Professional Writing in Kinesiology and Sports Medicine

Professional Writing in Kinesiology and Sports Medicine

Mark Knoblauch, PhD, LAT, ATC, CSCS
Clinical Assistant Professor
University of Houston
Houston, Texas

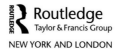
Routledge
Taylor & Francis Group

NEW YORK AND LONDON

Cover Artist: Lori Shields

First published in 2019 by SLACK Incorporated

Published 2024 by Routledge
605 Third Avenue, New York, NY 10158

and by Routledge
4 Park Square, Milton Park, Abingdon, Oxon OX14 4RN

Routledge is an imprint of the Taylor & Francis Group, an informa business

Library of Congress Cataloging-in-Publication Data

Names: Knoblauch, Mark, editor.
Title: Professional writing in kinesiology and sports medicine / [edited by]
  Mark Knoblauch.
Description: Thorofare, NJ : Slack Incorporated, [2019] | Includes
  bibliographical references and index.
Identifiers: LCCN 2018050873 (print)|ISBN 9781630915063(paperback)
Subjects: | MESH: Medical Writing | Kinesiology, Applied | Sports Medicine
Classification: LCC R119 (print) | NLM WB 890 | DDC
  808.06/661--dc23
LC record available at https://lccn.loc.gov/2018050873

ISBN:9781630915063(pbk)
ISBN: 9781003526001(ebk)

DOI: 10.4324/9781003526001

Dedication

For DO and MC, to show what can happen when you take the time to mentor someone who needs a little extra help.

Contents

Acknowledgments

This textbook was a collaboration. Therefore, it requires a special thanks from myself as the editor to each of the contributing authors who took time out of their hectic schedules over the past year to develop the outstanding chapters in this book. It is rare that a book production schedule is adhered to, yet the 15 other authors involved in this project met each deadline without fail. It is because of their efforts that this book became a reality.

Because book writing can be a time-consuming ordeal, the families and loved ones of each contributing author also deserve a special thanks for being accepting of the time, effort, and sometimes even frustration involved with allowing each author to get their chapter "just right." Furthermore, as each author brings his or her own unique writing perspective, it would be remiss to not also acknowledge those mentors instrumental in developing each chapter author's writing talents and perspectives over the years.

Personally, I want to thank every colleague of mine who offered support, encouragement, and guidance along the journey from moving this book from concept to completion. I also want to acknowledge my family for putting up with the numerous "Daddy's on his computer again" moments required of many evenings, weekends, and holiday breaks in order to keep this book moving forward.

Finally, I want to thank the publisher, SLACK Incorporated, for being accepting of my vision for this project and giving it the chance to succeed.

About the Editor

Mark Knoblauch, PhD, LAT, ATC, CSCS is a clinical assistant professor and clinical coordinator of the Master of Athletic Training Program at the University of Houston. He has been certified as an athletic trainer for more than 20 years and has worked clinically at both the university and junior college level. Mark received his PhD in Kinesiology from the University of Houston and completed a post-doctoral fellowship in Molecular Physiology and Biophysics from Baylor College of Medicine, where his research focus was on skeletal muscle damage and signaling mechanisms. He is a member of the National Athletic Trainers' Association (NATA), National Strength and Conditioning Association, and the Southwest Athletic Trainers' Association (SWATA), and is a site visitor for the Commission on Accreditation of Athletic Training Education. As a professional, he has been involved with several committees for the NATA and SWATA, including serving as Chair of the Research and Education Foundation's Student Writing Contests as well as Chair of The SWATA Free Communication and Research Committee.

Contributing Authors

Rehal Bhojani, MD, FAAFP, CAQSM
(Chapter 10)
Sports Medicine Physician
Memorial Hermann Medical Group
Houston, Texas

Craig R. Denegar, PhD, PT, ATC, FNATA
(Chapter 8)
Professor, Director of Doctor of Physical
Therapy Program
University of Connecticut
Storrs, Connecticut

Jon Gray, EdD (Chapter 4)
Instructional Associate Professor
University of Houston
Houston, Texas

Jay Hertel, PhD, ATC, FACSM, FNATA
(Chapter 8)
Joe H. Gieck Professor of Sports Medicine
University of Virginia
Charlottesville, Virginia

Jeff G. Konin, PhD, ATC, PT, FACSM, FNATA
(Chapter 14)
Vice President for Global Education &
Research
American Institute of Balance
American Institute for Continuing Medical
Education
Largo, Florida

Laura Kunkel, EdD, LAT, ATC, PES (Chapter 9)
Clinical Associate Professor
University of Texas at Arlington
Arlington, Texas

Mitzi S. Laughlin, PhD, LAT, ATC
(Chapters 2, 5)
Chief Scientist
Fondren Orthopedic Research Institute
Houston, Texas

Melissa Long, EdD, LAT, ATC, PES, LMT, CMT
(Chapter 3)
Assistant Professor
Abilene Christian University
Abilene, Texas

Thomas Lowder, PhD (Chapter 11)
Assistant Professor
University of Central Arkansas
Conway, Arkansas

Sarah A. Manspeaker, PhD, LAT, ATC
(Chapter 12)
Assistant Professor
Duquesne University
Pittsburgh, Pennsylvania

Jennifer M. Medina McKeon, PhD, ATC, CSCS
(Chapter 13)
Assistant Professor
Ithaca College
Ithaca, New York

Patrick O. McKeon, PhD, ATC, CSCS
(Chapter 1)
Associate Professor
Ithaca College
Ithaca, New York

Elisabeth C. Rosencrum, PhD, NH-LAT,
ATC, CSCS (Chapter 14)
Assistant Professor
Athletic Training
Department of Health and Human
Performance
Health and Human Enrichment Cluster
Plymouth State University
Plymouth, New Hampshire

Luzita Vela, PhD, LAT, ATC (Chapter 15)
Assistant Professor of Education
University of Virginia
Charlottesville, Virginia

Josh Yellen, EdD, LAT, ATC (Chapter 7)
Director
Master of Athletic Training Program
Department of Health and
    Human Performance
University of Houston
Houston, Texas

Preface

Welcome to *Professional Writing in Kinesiology and Sports Medicine*. As editor, I am excited to present this textbook to students and professionals in the fields of Kinesiology and Sports Medicine as both a guide and a resource for improving their professional writing.

Professional writing is supposed to be relatively straightforward. As researchers, we write the manuscript and it gets published; that's the plan. American pugilist Mike Tyson famously stated, "Everyone has a plan until they get punched in the mouth." For any researcher who has ever submitted for publication what he or she felt was an outstanding manuscript, getting a scathing manuscript critique back from peer review probably felt a lot like a figurative punch in the mouth. Even worse is when the reviewer's comments expose a convoluted mix of sentences and thoughts that were not evident in the final draft. It is times like those that we often choose to blame the reviewer for not looking at the work with an open mind. Rather, we may need to take a step back and recognize that our writing was simply not clear enough.

Similarly, we may often see an older version of our own writing in drafts generated by students. It is not uncommon to see a subsequent lack of flow in the sentences and paragraphs, or perhaps a few excessively wordy sentences. For many students, their first introduction to professional or scientific writing may come from their primary investigator's request for a literature review or a class case study. In reviewing available texts that I could recommend for assisting students with their professional writing, I found that the majority of textbooks centered on writing examples heavily immersed in basic science techniques. I felt that this emphasis on basic science presented a sort of disconnect with students and professionals in clinical-based research, which in turn helped me recognize the need for a writing textbook focused on clinical-based Kinesiology and Sports Medicine.

For that reason, I moved to develop a text that encompasses all of what I felt students and professionals in the fields of Kinesiology and Sports Medicine could benefit from. These 2 fields encompass a wide variety of career paths including Exercise Science, Physical Therapy, and Athletic Training, among many others. As these fields continue to incorporate the model of evidence-based medicine, the need for professionals to prepare, disseminate, and understand high-quality research becomes paramount. Furthermore, with fields such as Athletic Training now moving toward joining other established fields that require a graduate degree to enter the profession, an increased curricular focus on research ensures that students will need a thorough and practical guide to help them improve their professional writing.

Therefore, this book is designed to serve as a resource for students and professionals in the fields of Kinesiology and Sports Medicine to improve their professional writing skills. To accomplish this goal, the book has been roughly organized into 3 sections. Section I consists of Chapters 1 to 5 and focuses on the foundational concepts of professional writing. Here, the reader is first exposed in Chapter 1 to how writing conveys thought, and details how effective writing skills can be a valuable asset to a writer. Next, the foundational components of successful writing are discussed in subsequent chapters, detailing how to develop a quality outline, followed by how to choose the most effective words when writing, and closing with how to draft strong sentences and paragraphs.

Section II consists of Chapters 6 to 10 and focuses on what may be considered the "meat" of professional academic writing—the manuscript. This section starts with a chapter that walks the reader through the guidelines that all submitted manuscripts must adhere to—the journal's *Author's Guide*. Next are chapters that use concepts from Section I to help the reader develop attention-grabbing titles and abstracts, followed by how to draft a strong research manuscript and case report. The final chapter of Section II outlines the intricacies of the various subheadings that exist in some journals such as a Conclusion or Uniqueness section.

Because funding a quality scientific study as well as presenting the findings requires unique writing techniques, Section III consists of Chapters 11 to 15 and focuses on these ancillary aspects of professional writing. The section then addresses ethical issues related to professional writing, such as plagiarism and copyright, before closing with a chapter focusing on how to help relieve the stress of writing.

This book brings together a collection of experts well-versed on professional writing in the fields of Kinesiology and Sports Medicine. In each chapter they outline concepts that draw from their own experiences to help the reader become more competent in his or her own professional writing. Because professional writing can be difficult and even frustrating at times, it is the intent of all chapter authors that the material in this book help students, as well as professionals, become more productive and more efficient at their own writing. We wish you all the best of luck in the pursuit of science as well as in your writing.

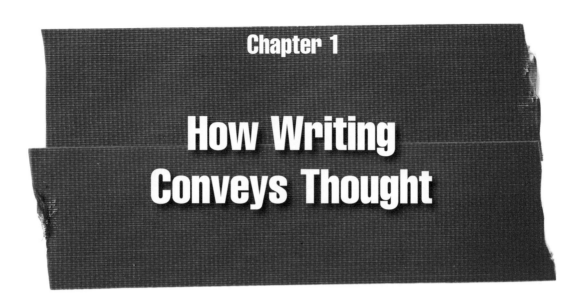

Chapter 1

How Writing Conveys Thought

Patrick O. McKeon, PhD, ATC, CSCS

Writing is a form of communication that is critically important to humans. It provides a means to capture thoughts and convey them to others. As well, it affords the ability to reflect on what an individual's or particular group's thoughts and perceptions were at certain points in history. Looking back at primitive petroglyphs or hieroglyphs across the world, one can get a sense of what prehistoric ancestors tens of thousands of years ago experienced in their daily lives. Writing has afforded humans the ability to catalog thoughts in a way that others can build on and advance as a species to solve some of the world's most complex problems. Whether it was anticipating animal migrations, charting the stars, or understanding love and affection, writing provides the opportunity to engage in a richly human experience.

The focus of this chapter is on scientific writing. This form of writing is used to convey particular thoughts, insights, and knowledge to a broader audience based on a systematic process of gathering and interpreting information. It is critically important for both the writer and reader to understand the systematic approach of science and its dissemination to its intended readership. Scientific dissemination is the cornerstone of scientific knowledge; therefore, clarity is its critical feature. To write scientifically is to engage in a practice that dates back to Aristotle and links all of the great scientists in history. In this chapter, the structural and functional elements of scientific writing to convey thought will be discussed, but first it is important to understand what science is and where it came from.

A Very Brief History of Science

When we use the term *science* today, a sense of authority comes to mind. It is used to highlight the certainty of an idea based on a systematic process carried out by scientists. In the media, writers and reporters bombard consumers with information validated by "science." It is apparent that the word carries a great deal of influence, but what actually is science? To understand the nature of scientific writing, it is first important to understand its origins.

Knoblauch M. *Professional Writing in Kinesiology and Sports Medicine* (pp 1-12).

The pursuit of science first began with Aristotle. He brought forth the idea to use a particular system of thought and observation to uncover underlying truths about nature and the universe. This process, known as *syllogism*, provided a framework for comparing what we see in reality to the potential underlying truths that govern it. Through careful development of premises (sentences used to affirm or deny the existence of a particular phenomenon), he looked for consistencies among observations in reality and began to formulate a sense of truth about the particular phenomena observed. Aristotle named the knowledge developed from this line of reasoning *Episteme*, which means "knowledge" in Greek.

The key feature of the knowledge derived from Episteme was that it could be demonstrated and replicated by others. A good example of this was his underlying truth that the Earth was the center of the universe and all objects on Earth had their natural resting place closest to the center. If one picked up a rock and threw it, the rock would return to Earth, which Aristotle considered the natural resting place of all forms (as close to the center of the Earth as possible). Aristotle was able to demonstrate this repeatedly with all different types of material and others were able to replicate his findings. The consistency of his observations and that others could replicate them led to this becoming scientific knowledge. By demonstrating and replicating these events, Aristotle found that he could not only explain why objects moved the way they did but also predict how objects would behave in the future. Therefore, knowledge is the purposeful linking of relevant information to develop meaning. Meaning then becomes the ability to explain and/or predict a phenomenon. The systematic process Aristotle developed became known as the *instrument* (another name is *method*) by which scientific knowledge was created. In Greek, instrument translates to "Organon." The Organon became the authoritative text of scientific thought. From this method, the notion that the Earth was the center of the universe and all objects seek their natural resting place closest to the center stood as a sound theory for almost 1800 years!

Based on Aristotle's system, there were 2 component parts to science: theory and observation. A theory is a general principle about an underlying truth that governs particular phenomena. An observation is an individual experience at one moment in relation to that phenomenon. Aristotle used theories and observations interdependently in Episteme. If starting with a theory, one might postulate what a future observation in reality might be. This form of reasoning became known as *deduction*. In deductive reasoning, a scientist starts with a theory, a generalization derived from previous knowledge as to what might be considered an underlying truth to what governs a phenomenon, and then observes what occurs in reality. Such reasoning works as follows:

Theory: All football players are male.

Observation: Chris is a football player.

Deductive conclusion: Chris is male.

In this example, Chris might or might not actually be male. If Chris is actually female, then the entire theory that all football players are male is incorrect. Therefore, a major issue for deductive reasoning is that if a single observation made does not agree with the original theory, the observer must abandon the theory.

Inductive reasoning is the opposite of deductive reasoning. This type of reasoning starts with a series of observations in which the observer looks for commonalities among them. By systematically evaluating these observations for common trends, the observer can develop propositions about the underlying truth governing the phenomenon observed. Upon reaching consistency within observations, a hypothesis is generated about how the next observation would likely behave. If the next observation falls in line with previous observations, the hypothesis is validated. If the observation fails to follow the proposition, the hypothesis is falsified and future observations must continue in order to explore other elements that may contribute to a better understanding of the underlying truth. From Aristotle, we learned that careful and systematic observations of phenomena could take on great meaning (ie, lead to an ability to explain and predict the phenomena encountered in nature). Critical to this process was the ability to connect a proposition to relevant evidence and draw logical conclusions. Many of the ideas brought forth by Aristotle through his epistemological reasoning led to great advancements in human understanding, and his method was the cornerstone of scientific knowledge until the Enlightenment.

The Scientific Revolution

In the 16th and 17th centuries, throughout the Enlightenment, the methodological scrutiny of observations became the centerpiece of knowledge derived from Episteme. Two of the most influential thinkers during that time, Francis Bacon and Rene Descartes, challenged Aristotle's Organon because the conclusions drawn from it were based on the combination of observations, preconceived assumptions, and previous knowledge of the observer. Bacon developed a new instrument (*Novum Organum* in Latin) for knowledge based on Aristotle's foundation and referred to it as *Scientia*, or knowledge, in Latin. The process of developing knowledge through observations then got its modern name: science! Bacon and his contemporaries, including Galileo, Newton, Locke, Descartes, and many others, believed that one's senses, prior experiences, and preconceived expectations can play tricks on the ability to correctly and consistently observe the world. The observer may have preconceived biases about what future observations "should" be and therefore rely on these preconceived notions rather than actual observations to draw conclusions about an underlying truth. Therefore, in order to reduce bias in scientific observations, the observer must be objective (neutral to and disinterested) in the outcome from a personal standpoint. *Objectivity* refers to the ability to observe systematically free of any preconceived notions of the outcome. It was the work of Bacon and many others during the Enlightenment that would later form the contemporary scientific method. The hallmark of this method was the disinterested nature of scientists. Based on their objectivity, they were free to explore the great questions of nature without being connected to a particular outcome. While contemporary scientists have scrutinized whether scientists can truly be disinterested, it still represents the method by which scientists should interpret the answers to the questions they raise.

Throughout the development of science known today, there is one thing that links all of the methods, theories, observations, and advancements together: the written word. From Aristotle to Bacon to Francis Collins, it is the ability to convey in writing the theories, observations, and their subsequent interpretations that enhances the human endeavor called *science*. Writing scientifically is a means of sharing observations and critical information for demonstration and replication by others to uncover the truth about what governs the phenomena encountered in nature. In order to engage in it meaningfully, there are certain rules that must be followed. In the next section of this chapter, the characteristics of scientific writing will be discussed that make it … well … scientific.

The Importance of Communication as a Means of Advancing Science

Science is a human endeavor that shapes the way scientists communicate meaningfully with one another and with the public. Therefore, science rests on a foundation of sound and meaningful communication. The medium of this communication is the written word. In order to be useful, it must be readily accessible to others. A scientist may uncover the most important of universal truths, but if he or she cannot communicate it effectively to others, it is meaningless (no ability to explain and/or predict). Science, by its nature, needs to be generalizable beyond the original observations that derived it. Therefore, a critical job of the scientific writer is to transform highly technical information about the reasoning, methods, and results of this systematic process into a digestible form for larger audiences without corrupting the original insights gained.

With this in mind, scientific writing is one of the most challenging forms of writing that there is. Most students and scholars become overwhelmed when embarking on sharing their findings with others based on the intimidating act of expressing ideas that are meaningful to a larger

Sidebar 1-1

Questions to ask when selecting words:

1. Is the reader going to understand this word? If not, is an operational definition needed?
2. Are the word choices the most accurate to convey the meaning?
3. Are specific word choices adding to the clarity of a particular thought?

audience while maintaining the components necessary to reproduce the results found. Before we move toward the essential elements of scientific writing, a review of some of the foundational elements of writing in its purest form is needed. Science stands on the foundation of writing.

From Words to Paragraphs: The Structural Elements of Scientific Writing

Writing begins with words. Words can be linked into a sentence. Sentences can be linked into a paragraph. Paragraphs can be linked into a thesis. Sounds simple, but this can be a very overwhelming process. While a person readily recognizes words in his or her own language, it is important to step back and recognize the role words play in communication. A word is a group of letters. Letters are symbols connoting certain sounds. When linked together, these letters can convey a particular meaning. When reading in a first language, we may take for granted the power of words. However, when reading a language that is unfamiliar, it becomes apparent that, while the grouping of letters may have the same meaning, it is unrecognizable to the reader, and therefore meaningless. Episteme and Scientia are good examples of this idea. Both mean "knowledge," but use different letters. Science incorporates a language in and of itself. Many of the words used may be specific to a particular discipline of science. With this in mind, word choices and their operational definitions play a large role in communicating thoughts effectively.

Word Choices and Operational Definitions

When writing, clarity is the most important goal. Often, there exists the temptation to sound more "scientific" by using bigger words, such as extrapolate (to generalize) or concatenate (to link together). While this may enhance a writer's ego, it may not serve the reader well who is trying to digest the information presented. Instead, writers should choose words that are accurate, simple to understand, and meaningful to the intended audience. Accuracy means that the words actually communicate the thought the writer is trying to convey. Simplicity refers to the ability to make it easy for the reader to understand the thought. Meaningful indicates that both the writer and reader have the ability to explain and/or predict the ideas expressed with the word.

Meaning is an important factor in choosing words so that both the writer and reader understand their use in explanation or prediction. If there is a word that may have more than one meaning, it is important to define the word for the reader in how the writer intends to use it. By operationally defining a word or phrase for the reader and choosing the simplest words to communicate his or her thoughts accurately, a writer can ensure that thoughts are conveyed meaningfully to the reader (Sidebar 1-1).

Sidebar 1-2

Questions to ask when developing good sentences:

1. What thought is the writer attempting to communicate to the reader?
2. Does the writer use active voice to clearly articulate the relationship between the subject and object?
3. Does the writer have more than one thought in this sentence? If so, can the sentence be split into at least 2 to more effectively communicate the thought to the reader?

Sentence Structure and Voice

Sentences are words linked together to communicate a single idea. While this sounds like a straightforward lesson from elementary school, as an editor of a journal, I often see component parts of sentences missing. Sentences minimally contain an actor (the subject), the action or state of being of the actor (a verb), and the thing acted upon (the object). There are other component parts of sentences, but these are the most relevant features to focus on. When constructing sentences, it is important to write actively. Put the subject at the center of the action and the object as the result. This is referred to as *active voice*. Here is an example:

> *The investigator conducted several experiments.* (5 words)

In this case, the investigator is the subject, conducted is the action in past tense, and several experiments was the object of the sentence. There is a tendency for writers to mix these up, such as:

> *Several experiments were conducted by the researcher.* (7 words)

In this case, the object (several experiments) came before the subject. This is referred to as *passive voice*. Passive voice emphasizes the object and de-emphasizes the subject. As well, in order to write passively, more words are needed. When writing simplistically and accurately, the less words the better. Therefore, to enhance the clarity, simplicity, and accuracy of sentences, write in active voice.

Another factor associated with sentence formation is the thought conveyed. Ideally, one sentence contains one thought. If a sentence contains more than one thought, it becomes difficult to grasp the intended meaning. For example:

> *Chronic ankle instability is a condition marked by repeated episodes of giving way after an initial ankle sprain. Several factors including impaired postural control, improper gait mechanics, and diminished strength of the periarticular muscles increase the risk of developing chronic ankle instability.*

Within these 2 sentences, clear thoughts are expressed. The first sentence indicates the key features of the condition, and the second sentence indicates contributing factors for it.

Contrast those 2 sentences to this one:

> *Chronic ankle instability, a condition marked by repeated episodes of giving way, has been linked to several factors for its development, including impaired postural control, improper gait mechanics, and diminished strength; all of which have been shown to increase the risk of its development.*

While the writer provided the reader with same information, it is difficult to discern the thoughts expressed. A writer can form effective sentences by carefully evaluating the word choices, the voice (active vs passive), and whether the thoughts are conveyed clearly to the reader (Sidebar 1-2).

Paragraph Formation—From Topic to Conclusion

A paragraph is a group of sentences linked together to communicate an idea that is composed of several thoughts. A writer uses each sentence to communicate a single thought. When combined, multiple sentences (thoughts) can effectively communicate an idea (a group of thoughts purposefully linked together). To formulate an effective paragraph, 3 essential elements are needed: (1) a topic sentence, (2) supporting sentences, and (3) a concluding sentence.

The topic sentence communicates the overarching thought to the reader on the idea of the paragraph. The supporting sentences then serve to provide the evidence for the topic. The concluding sentence then serves to tie together the supporting sentences in the context of the topic. These should flow in order for ease of reading. An example is as follows:

> *Chronic ankle instability affects many different physically active populations.(TOPIC) In recent epidemiological studies, investigators found that 45% of athletes who suffered an initial ankle sprain in high school went on to develop recurrent issues 5 years later. (SUPPORT) This trend was also observed in the collegiate level in which 52% of all athletes who suffered an ankle sprain went on to suffer subsequent sprains.(SUPPORT) Likewise, in the military, 47% of noncombat-related ankle sprain patients continued to complain of persistent instability symptoms over a 5-year period.(SUPPORT) Therefore, chronic ankle instability is a pervasive issue in those who are physically active and suffer an ankle sprain.(CONCLUSION)*

While this example appears to be clear, writers may have a difficult time choosing the appropriate topic and ensuring unity throughout the supporting sentences. A lack of topic can lead to a lack of conclusion in a paragraph. Here is an example along the same vein:

> *In recent epidemiological studies, investigators found that 45% of athletes who suffered an initial ankle sprain in high school went on to develop recurrent issues 5 years later. Some patients demonstrate dorsiflexion deficits with asymmetries up to 2 cm. As well, others have reported postural control deficits in those with chronic ankle instability. Still others also report high functional limitations and participation restrictions in this population.*

In this example, there are well-developed sentences that communicate distinct thoughts. However, no clear topic links them together. Because of the absence of a topic sentence, there is also no ability to draw a conclusion. This is a very short example. Often, writers may extend paragraphs to 10 to 15 sentences not clearly linked and fill up an entire page with a paragraph. The burden then falls on the reader to discern the relationships among the thoughts, how they may or may not communicate an overall topic. When constructing paragraphs, developing a sense of the most important ideas to communicate first is critical. Chapters 4 and 5 will focus more extensively on sentence and paragraph development and how to clearly articulate an idea (Sidebar 1-3).

From Paragraphs to Thesis: The Functional Elements of Forming an Argument

Good writing skills center on the essential elements for building an argument and helping the reader capture what the writer is trying to say. This process, known as *rhetoric*, was first developed by Aristotle and continues to influence how writing, especially scientific writing, is carried out today. As stated earlier, science is only as good as its generalizability to a larger audience. There are 3 elements to rhetoric: ethos, logos, and pathos.

Ethos: Establishing a Writer's Credibility in the Reader's Eyes

Ethos pertains to the authority and character of the writer. The key issue with ethos in writing is the ability for the writer to demonstrate expertise in the content area of interest. Based on word choices, sentence structure, paragraph development, and content details, a reader can gain a sense of the quality of information presented. If a reader cannot easily extract and comprehend the content and context of the writer, the ethos of the writer can be called into question. Originally, letters were the accepted form of communication between scientists. These letters provided a framework to discuss findings of relevant studies and the context of these findings in the larger body of knowledge about them. Because scientists wrote letters to each other and the quality of their shared works, their ethos was inherently established.

Since the dawn of the first scientific journal from the Royal Society of London in 1660, thousands of scientific journals have emerged with broader public readership. Scientific writing no longer centers on being able to communicate effectively with colleagues who are familiar with one's work and area of expertise. Establishing ethos in scientific writing is far more challenging. A scientific writer must build a case for the knowledge contribution using established literature from the past to guide current research questions. If the writer cannot build a clear case for the science presented, the ethos of the writer is diminished in the reader's eyes.

A critical factor in establishing ethos in scientific writing is the use of existing scientific literature effectively. Throughout a manuscript, referring back to what is known, what remains unknown, and the potential for the unknown to become known all helps to establish the ethos of the writer. Consider the following statements:

> *Chronic ankle instability was first established as a medical condition in 1965 by Freeman and colleagues who defined it as the tendency for the ankle to "give way" after an initial sprain. Since then, numerous investigators have attempted to capture the contributing factors to this phenomenon. Key factors consistently identified from these investigations include impaired postural control, improper gait mechanics, and diminished strength of periarticular muscles.*

Contrast the above statements with the following:

> *Chronic ankle instability is a condition where the ankle has a tendency to "give way." There have been several factors identified that may contribute to it; however, it remains unclear which factors are most important.*

While much of the information in both sets of statements are similar, the first provides the reader with a sense that the writer is aware of the current state of evidence associated with chronic ankle instability and therefore has a sense of authority on the topic. The lack of specificity from the second set of statements reduces the possibility for the reader to see the writer as an authority on the topic. Through clearly articulated ethos, the scientific writer takes on the more significant role of scientific author (a writer who has established ethos, and therefore AUTHORity in the reader's eyes).

Logos: Constructing an Argument Based on Evidence

The second element of rhetoric in scientific writing is logos, which Aristotle defined as the ability to build an argument through sound reason. Key to logos is the ability to guide the reader in the process by which the writer purposefully links propositions and conclusions. Logos is used as a means to bring forth validity in a statement for the reader to see that a proposition is self-evident. When using logos in scientific writing, the writer appeals to the reader through reason and logic. Therefore, logos centers on the presentation of evidence to support a proposition, most often presented as figures and tables. Key pieces of evidence include data-driven examples (*P* values, mean differences, rate ratios, etc) that provide the reader with a sense of magnitude and consistency of the evidentiary support for a proposition. In this way, logos centers on the use of reasoning (eg, inductive or deductive) to link the propositions and conclusions. If there is no evidence to support a proposition, then it is simply a statement based on authority (ethos) to which no conclusion can be drawn.

Consider the following statements:

> *Chronic ankle instability is pervasive in soccer and basketball. In a recent large-scale systematic review, Attenborough et al[1] highlighted that out of all sports, soccer and basketball account for the highest number of participants with recurrent ankle sprains, 60% and 61%, respectively.*

The evidence presented supports the proposition that chronic ankle instability is pervasive in soccer and basketball. Logos then helps the reader see the inductive nature of the proposition that chronic ankle instability is pervasive based on the findings from multiple observations compiled within a systematic review. In this way, the reader can appreciate the authority of the writer to make such a proposition and see the logic in the argument that the proposition actually represents a self-evident truth. Where there is no evidence, there is no sound argument. Writers often fall into the trap of simply providing a reference for the proposition as opposed to using logos to support it. Consider a statement like this:

> *Chronic ankle instability is pervasive in soccer and basketball.[1]*

This statement is based on the writer's ethos. While the writer provided a reference for the statement, there is actually no logos associated with it. Instead, the onus falls on the reader to verify that the reference is actually related to the statement. In addition, it is then up to the reader to sift through the entire separate referenced publication for relevant findings to support the proposition. Either the reader must buy into the ethos of the writer or critically examine the use of evidence found in the external reference to inductively or deductively support the proposition. This can be exhausting for the reader!

Ethos and logos play off of one another in the development of a paragraph. As discussed earlier, a paragraph consists of a topic sentence, supporting sentences, and a concluding sentence. Through the lens of ethos and logos, the topic sentence transforms into the proposition based on the ethos of the writer and the supporting sentences transform into the logos to support it. The concluding sentence can then be used to guide the reader to see the link between the logos used and the proposition presented.

Pathos: Connecting to the Reader Emotionally

The third component of rhetoric centers on effectively communicating with the intended readership. Aristotle described pathos as the ability to establish and manipulate an emotional connection with one's audience. By understanding the hopes, needs, and experiences of the readership, a writer can tailor the message accordingly. Similar to ethos and logos, writers use pathos strategically to build the case for the impact scientific knowledge and the interpretation of its findings have on readers' lives and the greater society. Consider the following statements:

Sidebar 1-4

Questions to ask when developing a rhetorical argument:

Ethos

1. Has the writer established the relevant background to clearly articulate that he or she is an authority on the subject presented?

2. Are the propositions made by the writer in the context of the relevant background?

3. What is the intention of the writer for communicating the proposition?

Logos

1. What type of evidence does the writer need to support the proposition?

2. Does the use of evidence help the reader to grasp the proposition as self-evident?

3. What is the best way to present the evidence to the reader? As a table, figure, in text?

Pathos

1. Who is the target audience for the written communication?

2. Are there specific considerations for the method of communication that will help the writer develop an emotional connection with the reader?

3. Does the use of pathos help the reader gauge the importance of the writer's propositions?

Chronic ankle instability is pervasive in soccer and basketball. While ankle sprains are often considered benign in sport, patients with chronic ankle instability become trapped in a continuum of disability that leads to decreased physical activity, lower quality of life, and increased medical costs across their life span. It is imperative that we strive to enhance the recognition of the burden that these injuries carry with them, their substantial biopsychosocial consequences, and their impact on a person's quality of life.

The first statement was the original proposition stated earlier. What follows are statements that appeal to the reader's emotional concern for those who sprain their ankles in soccer and basketball and the lifelong struggles that may result. There is no logos presented here. Instead, the writer is attempting to connect with the reader on an emotional level. Similar to a lawyer appealing to the emotions of a jury, pathos is used to draw the reader into the writer's argument. Consequently, the writer must be perceptive to the hopes and desires of the readership for pathos to be effective.

The emotional connection is highly dependent on the familiarity of the reader to the clinical condition. Considering the statement above, if the reader is a physical therapist who works most commonly with stroke patients experiencing extreme functional losses in a very short time with little chance of recovery, his or her emotional connection with chronic ankle instability may be very weak. Comparatively, if the reader is an athletic trainer or physical therapist who has commonly seen patients drop out of sports participation due to ankle sprains, there may be a strong emotional connection. Therefore, pathos is highly dependent on the perspective of the reader.

Scientific writers must often check their ability to draw on the emotional connection with a broader public readership and limit the pathos incorporated into their arguments. Pathos is deemphasized based on the reader's expectation that scientists should have a disinterested viewpoint to their work as part of their ethos (eg, "just the facts, ma'am"). Disinterestedness is a quality that is expected in the development, collection, and analysis of data from a research study, but not necessarily for effective communication. A scientific writer can help the reader to engage in the discourse developed by drawing the reader into what is important to him or her. When using pathos as a rhetorical strategy, it is important then to be familiar with the intended audience and their expectations for scientific writing (Sidebar 1-4).

Figure 1-1. The dynamic interplay among the structural and functional elements of scientific writing. The structural elements (word choice, sentence structure, and paragraph formation) provide the foundation for building an argument. The functional elements (ethos, logos, and pathos) provide the contextual framework for the argument. It is essential to understand when developing an argument in scientific writing to work through both the structural and functional elements. The use and impact are dependent on the goal and nature of the written communication.

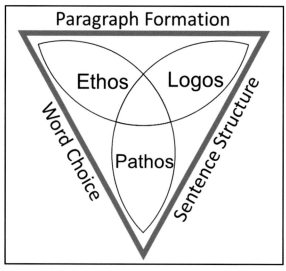

Understanding how and when to use combinations of ethos, logos, and pathos in scientific writing can enhance a writer's ability to effectively formulate and communicate scientific arguments (Figure 1-1). Word choice, sentence structure, and paragraph formation play critical roles in the argument's structure. The functional interplay among ethos, logos, and pathos then guides the content of the structure. By capitalizing on the functional and structural aspects of writing, a writer can build sound scientific arguments that help to advance the body of knowledge in a particular field. Without effective communication strategies, no matter how self-evident the findings, if a reader cannot discern the thoughts of the writer, the knowledge is meaningless (Sidebar 1-5).

Conclusion

Writing is a fundamental form of communication within science. By understanding and exploiting the structural and functional elements of scientific writing, a writer has the ability to influence a reader in the importance of the knowledge communicated. Word selection, sentence structure, and paragraph formation are the key structural elements of communication. The functional elements of developing effective arguments center on ethos, logos, and pathos. Writers communicate thought effectively to readers through the dynamic interplay between these structural and functional elements. Throughout the rest of this book, the contextual aspects of using these elements for developing scientific manuscripts will be presented. By having a clear understanding of how to communicate effectively with readers, writers can better construct effective writing strategies.

Sidebar 1-5

The Importance of Multiple Drafts

Communicating thought through the written word isn't easy. Having served as a reviewer, associate editor, and editor-in-chief of scientific journals, I spend much of my time and effort helping authors develop their ability to articulate their thoughts and arguments clearly for the reader. While I have gained a great deal of experience in writing because of this, my greatest lesson in writing came from my mother very early in my writing career— elementary school. She was a history major in college and viewed the written word as a means of not only communicating thought, but also cataloging human experience. To do so, ideas needed to be honed so that others could grasp them.

In my early academic career, I was a procrastinator. (Many might argue that I still am, but I haven't gotten around to proving them wrong yet.) Waiting often to complete writing assignments the night before they were due, I would struggle with what, how, and why to write. My mother would always ask to see my work and provide a thorough review of it before she would allow me to turn it in to the teacher. I would hand her my writing assignment thinking that I had captured all of the hopes and dreams of my teacher with my writing prowess. After several minutes of crossing out, writing margin comments, and underlining areas where my writing was not clear, she would hand my literary masterpiece back to me, say it was a good "first draft," and I needed to revise and resubmit to her. In her comments, she would often indicate that my paragraphs lacked grammatical structure and no clear topic, support, or concluding sentences. In short, my first draft was a free-flowing stream of consciousness as opposed to a well-articulated argument.

After multiple revisions, often late into the night (my mother is a saint) I would finally present a revised writing assignment that satisfied her standard. Upon turning it in to my teacher, I would often receive feedback that reinforced my mother's writing lesson. My teachers would comment that my writing was well developed and clearly organized. When returning home to present these results to my mother, she would highlight the importance of multiple drafts to ensure clarity of thought and purpose in writing. I continued the above process with my mother's help many times throughout middle school, high school, and my undergraduate work. Despite my immediate frustrations with the process, her lesson has been a beacon for me in my professional writing career.

When writing, be sure to afford enough time and effort for multiple drafts and the opportunity to scrutinize the structural and functional elements of your writing. Whether it be an essay, a scientific manuscript, or even a professional email, I find providing time for reflection and revision is critical for ensuring the clarity of my written communication. I guarantee that my first attempt is NOT my best attempt. In today's culture, I see the detriment of people firing off written comments on social media with no filter or reflection on their thoughts. This often leads to misinterpretation of ideas, public apologies, and loss of character. Taking time to think about what I want to say (my purpose in writing) has enhanced my ability to use ethos, logos, and pathos appropriately and effectively. Even more important is my mother's lesson to reflect and revise my writing to make sure that my word choices, sentence structure, and paragraph formation clearly articulate my thoughts and argument. My mother helped me see the value of the thinking, writing, reflecting, and revising process to capitalize on the structural and functional elements of writing. I urge the reader of this chapter to do the same. Thanks, Mom!

Bibliography

Aristotle, McKeon RP. *The Basic Works of Aristotle*. New York, NY: Random House; 1941.

Bredan AS, van Roy F. Writing readable prose: when planning a scientific manuscript, following a few simple rules has a large impact. *EMBO Rep*. 2006;7(9):846-849.

Butterfield H. *The Origins of Modern Science*. New York, NY: The Free Press; 1957.

Fahy K. Writing for publication: argument and evidence. *Women Birth*. 2008;21(3):113-117.

Fahy K. Writing for publication: the basics. *Women Birth*. 2008;21(2):86-91.

Gopen GD, Swan JA. The science of scientific writing. *American Scientist*. 1990;78(6):550-558.

Harmon JE, Gross AG. *The Scientific Literature: A Guided Tour*. Chicago, IL: The University of Chicago Press; 2007.

Johnson EM. The uses of the past: why science writers should care about the history of science and why scientists should too. *Scientific American*. https://blogs.scientificamerican.com/primate-diaries/uses-of-the-past/. Published January 17, 2012. Accessed June 11, 2018.

Knight KL, Ingersoll CD. Optimizing scholarly communication: 30 tips for writing clearly. *J Athl Train*. 1996;31(3):209-213.

Knight KL, Ingersoll CD. Structure of a scholarly manuscript: 66 tips for what goes where. *J Athl Train*. 1996;31(3):201-206.

McKeon PO, Medina McKeon JM, Geisler PR. Redefining professional knowledge in athletic training: whose knowledge is it anyway? *Athl Train Educ J*. 2017;12(2):95-105.

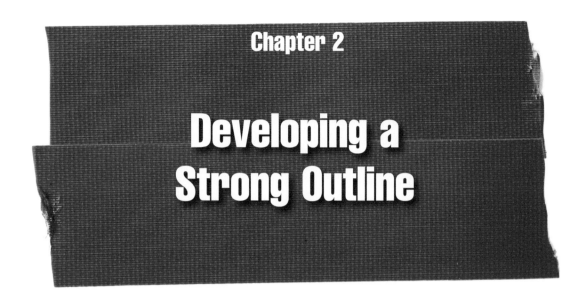

Chapter 2

Developing a Strong Outline

Mitzi S. Laughlin, PhD, LAT, ATC

As a salute to the proverbial high school English teacher, the importance of developing an outline prior to writing will be discussed in this chapter. In high school, most writers probably had to turn in an outline of a particular theme a week or so before the full paper was due. The teacher had valid reasons to require an outline. First of all, it required an organization of thoughts about the paper a week before it was due—no more last-minute procrastination. An outline also made the writer think through (minimally at least) the topic and organize his or her ideas. The outline also helped guide the writing and helped keep the writer on topic in order to prevent writing too much material that was ultimately deleted. So an outline was not just one more homework assignment, but it actually helped writers write better themes in high school English class and would also help when writing scientific manuscripts or creative works in the future.

Do I Really Need an Outline?

Many writers ask this question and the answer is the same whether they are a novice, seasoned writer, or somewhere in the middle. The answer is always YES, but the implementation of the outline may be different as more experience is gained as a writer. Readers of this textbook could be assumed to be novice or moderately experienced but still recognize a need for help with their writing. In this phase, a solid outline is a must before beginning to write sections of the manuscript, and it will pay off immensely at many other stages of writing.

First, writers should think of an outline as the skeleton of the overall scientific manuscript. It is the bones that holds everything together and allows for movement to the different parts. The outline should be brief but include all the parts of the paper—the topic, section headings, major sub-sections, and critical evidence to be presented. The outline moves from one part of the paper to the next in an organized manner so ideas are presented clearly to the reader. Since every section of the manuscript is represented in the outline, developing an outline requires writers to think through every section prior to writing the actual manuscript draft.

Knoblauch M. *Professional Writing in
Kinesiology and Sports Medicine* (pp 13-22).
© 2019 Taylor & Francis Group.

Sidebar 2-1

An outline …

- is the skeleton of the paper
- ensures you have thought through the topic
- gauges whether you have researched the topic thoroughly
- helps eliminate writer's block
- helps keep your writing on topic
- ultimately saves time

To organize their thoughts on the topic, writers should ask themselves "What do I want the reader to know when he or she finishes reading this manuscript?" Write down brief phrases that contain the main ideas of the topic. It is okay if it looks like a jumbled mess—just copy everything down including ideas, facts, phrases, and even key words.

During those times that writers totally draw a blank on their topic or only have a few scant ideas, they must recognize early on that they need to do more research or understand the topic better before trying to write. This is a key benefit of developing an outline prior to writing a manuscript. But beware of using "more research" as an excuse to justify procrastination. Review a few other relevant articles or a book chapter or two and then delve right back into the outline. Writers do not have to know every fact and reference that will be discussed at this stage but should be familiar with the focus and main ideas of each part of the manuscript.

Second, an outline helps get writers started and then helps them keep going once the writing begins. How many aspiring authors complain about writer's block and never get started actually writing? Spending a few minutes on an outline prevents this, as a writer who complains about writer's block is a writer who failed to outline. With an outline, writers have the topic and main ideas already organized and can get started writing on each section of the manuscript. This prevents having to stare at a blank screen saying "I don't have any words for this topic," as the focus and main ideas are already ready to go. Just start filling in the blanks linking one topic to the next and writer's block is long forgotten. Once into the act of writing, the outline sets the flow to continue writing and keep the writer on topic. By following the outline, writers are much less likely to veer off topic. This off-topic writing may be interesting but is eventually deleted from the manuscript or saved for a different project. Writers can save themselves time and words by staying on topic and following their outline (Sidebar 2-1).

Getting one's thoughts in order with an outline really does pay off. To see the difference, conduct an experiment by writing one manuscript with an outline and another without. In an overwhelming majority of cases the non-outline manuscript experience will be more frustrating and take more total time than the one that started with a solid outline.

Steps to Writing a Good Outline

Step 1: Gather Supplies

The first step in writing an outline is to gather the necessary supplies. There are many different tools that writers can choose from to write their outline. For most individuals, the supplies do not matter—just pick which one is most convenient and get started. Here are a few of the options, but there are many more:

- Paper and pen
- Word processor
- White board
- Sticky notes
- Index cards
- Evernote
- Mobile apps
- PowerPoint
- Poster board

Step 2: Formulate a Topic and Purpose Statement

A good outline requires a topic or reason to write the manuscript. The topic statement should be clear, concise, and be able to be fully developed within the limits of the manuscript. If the topic is too broad, the manuscript will be superficial and may not be able to cover all the main points to a sufficient depth. In this case, break it up into smaller pieces and save the list for future manuscripts (or grants). Pick one of the pieces to tackle as the first manuscript.

For a majority of scientific articles, the topic statement is written as "The purpose of this paper is … " and is in the last paragraph of the introduction, if not the last sentence. There are several common themes of scientific articles written on sports medicine topics:

- Educate patients
- Describe how to properly evaluate a condition
- Evaluate different treatment options
- Describe a case study of an unusual condition or unusual presentation of a common condition

Each of the above-mentioned themes could be describing the same condition such as patella tendinitis. A manuscript could educate the patient, describe how to evaluate patella tendinitis, evaluate whether ice or electrical stimulation was a better treatment option, or describe an unusual presentation of this common disorder. This is one general condition, but many different manuscripts can and have been written about patella tendinitis. So it is important for writers to know what they want to write about and more importantly what they do not want to write about, as well as what they want the reader to take away after reading the manuscript.

> ***The purpose of this study was to*** *determine how gender, age at injury, and activity level at injury affect the risk of an additional knee injury occurring in the time interval between ACL injury and reconstruction.*[1]

> ***The purpose of this study was to*** *evaluate preoperative and final follow-up shoulder function scores, mobility, satisfaction, and return to work in patients after reverse shoulder arthroplasty with a workers' compensation claim and to compare them with an age-, gender-, and diagnosis-matched control group without a workers' compensation claim.*[2]

Exercise 1

Organize the following study ideas into a purpose statement.

1. Girls, 12 to 15 years old, ACL prevention program and control, soccer teams, 2-season follow-up
2. Baseball pitchers, pitch counts related to shoulder and elbow injury rates, NCAA Division 1
3. Linemen (football players), comfort and stability of knee braces, Texas high schools

Step 3: Collect Evidence and Talking Points

Once the purpose of the study is clearly written, the next step is collecting evidence to help prove the main point and talking points that the writer wants the reader to take away from the article. This step is usually called *brainstorming* and can completed with any of the supplies mentioned in Step 1. The goal is to get all the ideas, possible references, and key words together in one place—the writing implement does not matter, so writers should use whatever supplies they are most comfortable with.

While brainstorming ideas, work to collect the following:

- Talking points
- Theories
- References
- Key words
- Key ideas
- Alternative theories

A review of one's clinical or laboratory notebook may be helpful to recall any ideas developed while performing the experiment. Also, a quick review of literature will produce a few ideas. Those are the more formal brainstorming sessions, but informal brainstorming produces ideas too. Ideas can come during random events, and writers need to be ready to jot them down (Sidebar 2-2).

At this point, the style of the collection does not matter—sentences, bullet points, names, key words, or all of the above are okay in the same collection. Once all the brainstormed components have been gathered initially, take an honest look at the collection. If writing a journal manuscript, the word count is usually somewhere between 3500 and 6000 words. Is the collection more than 150 bullet points? Maybe there is enough for more than one manuscript or there is a need to trim the collection a little before starting to organize them for the outline. But if writing a book chapter or a more creative work, 150 bullet points may be just perfect. What about when trying to write a journal manuscript and only 5 to 8 ideas have been generated? Unless these are major ideas with several subideas, it is time for more research. With a scant number of ideas, there is not enough material to write a full manuscript. In those cases, writers should save themselves some time later and do a little more research and review on their topic before continuing.

Once having developed a collection of ideas, it is time to group them into common themes. Read through each one, is there a common theme—by theory, treatment modality, injury severity, chronological order, etc? Once a first-level grouping of these ideas is complete, look to see if a second grouping could further organize the collection. Beware of "chronological order" as a grouping technique, as the resulting manuscript is often extremely boring and taxing for the reader.

Sidebar 2-2

Ideas have come to me in almost every aspect of daily life, but are more frequent for me when I am:

- Out on a run
- Taking a shower
- Waking up in the middle of the night

I have also collected all the material needed for a grant proposal during a walk across campus on a nice spring day (maybe several loops). Just remember ideas will come at all times during the day so be ready to capture them.

Step 4: Produce a Solid Outline

Outlines for Research Manuscripts

Most research journals have a standard style and are fairly linear in their presentation of ideas. The journal article starts at Step A and ends at Step F, passing sequentially through B – C – D – E to arrive at F. After one's topic sentence is written and ideas are organized into common themes, the next step to writing a good outline is to read the instructions to authors for the target journal. (See Chapter 6 for a detailed look into a journal's *Author Guide*.) Most journals have a set style and will provide the first level of the outline to manuscript authors.

- Introduction followed by purpose statement
- Methods
- Results
- Discussion
- Conclusions or Practical Application (some journals)

Depending on the focus of the journal, the first level of the outline may differ, but a majority of research journals adhere to this format. As such, each level of the outline and what types of information should be included in each level will be discussed.

Introduction

The Introduction section is sometimes also called *background*. This is the manuscript author's opportunity to grab the reader's interest so he or she keeps reading the rest of the paper. Additionally, the author will want to introduce the reader to the main topic and give the reader the relevant background information needed to understand the paper. After reading this section, all readers should be on the same page and know the same relevant facts. Remember the topic and purpose statement that were carefully crafted earlier? The Introduction section builds the topic to highlight the significance of the purpose statement.

Most Introduction or Background sections are 3 to 5 paragraphs maximum, so authors will need to be clear, concise, and present only the most relevant facts. The outline for this section is thus quite short. Here is a generic outline for the introduction:

1. Identify sports medicine condition
   a. Present general information on the condition
      i. Who it affects
      ii. What it is

      iii. When does it occur

      iv. Why or how does it occur

   b. Present evidence on the condition

      i.   Short-/long-term outcomes

      ii. Treatment costs and duration

      iii. Adverse outcomes

      iv. Possible new treatments

2. State what is unknown or problematic about this condition

   a. Why is this a problem

   b. What is unknown

   c. How this problem/new treatment may impact outcomes

3. Purpose statement

The entire Introduction section should build from the general to the specific and then to the purpose statement. With journals limiting word counts, the Introduction section is usually the first to be trimmed down. In the outline, use only the most relevant facts and save the others for the Discussion section.

Exercise 4

Review your list of brainstorming ideas from the last section. Which ones are suitable for the Introduction section? Write out the outline for the introduction. Are there any missing pieces?

Methods

The Methods section is also termed *Materials and Methods* in some journals. In a hypothesis-driven paper, this section is key to inform the readers about how the study was conducted. By reading the published article, the reader should be able to replicate the study in his or her own facility after reading and following the Methods section; however, this level of detail is not required for the outline. For many authors, the Methods section is fairly straightforward to outline and write. The major elements include:

1. Subjects

   a. Number, sex, age, height, weight

   b. Special characteristics, such as sport if subjects were selected from a particular sport

2. Experimental design

3. Procedures

4. Materials used

5. Statistical analysis

When using human or animal subjects, the information needed for the Methods section is usually written for the Institutional Review Board, Committee for the Protection of Human Subjects, or Institutional Animal Care and Use Committee application prior to performing the study. Therefore, when later organizing information for the manuscript, the main points of the methods are already outlined in the application document and a little editing is all that might be needed to reflect exactly what was performed in the study.

Results

The Results section typically induces anxiety for many authors. But if manuscript authors plan ahead of time, the writing is fairly direct and simply reports the results of the experiment. Not every observation or data point needs to be included, but the major outcomes of the study need to be presented. Save the explanation and comparison of the results to other studies for the Discussion section. This is the main error seen with novice authors, as the initial draft of the Results section looks "boring" or "too short" so material is added that really belongs in the Discussion section.

To outline the Results section, authors should go back and reread the statistical analysis section. Present the results for each analysis mentioned. For example, suppose a study is comparing 2 groups of patients who received a novel treatment and the standard treatment. The statistical analysis section was probably written to compare baseline characteristics of the groups to make sure they do not differ at the beginning of the study and then compare outcome measures between the 2 groups. The Results section outline could look like this:

1. Baseline measures, compare treatment groups
   a. Age, height, and weight (*t* test)
   b. Sex (chi-square test or Fisher's Exact test)
   c. Pain (*t* test)
   d. Range of motion (*t* test)
   e. Table 1—presentation of baseline measures by treatment groups
2. Baseline to final outcome measures, compare treatment groups
   a. Pain (repeated-measures ANOVA)
   b. Range of motion (repeated-measures ANOVA)
   c. Time until return to sport (*t* test)
   d. Patient satisfaction with treatment (*t* test)
   e. Table 2—presentation of baseline to final outcome measures by treatment groups

Most journals require the mean and standard deviation (or standard error) for each variable and *P* values for each comparison test performed. Writing this out in paragraph form quickly becomes a jumbled list of numbers. To meet the journal's requirement, use a couple of tables to list all the numbers and report in the text the results of only the major outcomes.

In summary, the Results section is a fairly straightforward section to outline and write, but it does take some practice until all authors are comfortable writing this section. Remember that the Results section reports the results. Save the commentary and discussion of the results for the Discussion section.

Discussion

The Discussion section is viewed by many as a difficult section to write. But when writers start with a clear idea of the required content, it becomes much easier to write. First, the Discussion section is used to interpret the findings of a study in light of other studies or theories found in the literature. Second, manuscript authors can describe the significance of their findings and explain any new insights about the research topic. Authors should explain to the reader how the study has moved the understanding of the research question forward from where it was started in the introduction. Overall, this can be a very powerful section of writing and demonstrate the author's ability as a researcher to think critically and integrate the results of multiple studies on the topic.

When outlining the Discussion section, it is vital to organize the presentation in a clear and logical manner. Authors should spend some extra time at this stage checking their logic and assumptions. A flaw in logic in the Discussion section can derail even the best study that presents novel and innovative results. For the Discussion section outline, authors should start by looking at their key research findings and providing the answer to the research question from their introduction. Next, they will want to generalize their results to the larger body of knowledge in the field. For the outline, it is not necessary to write down every point that is planned to be made, but rather, to list the articles and references planned to be used. Once the articles and references are listed, organize

Figure 2-1. Discussion section pyramid starting with the specific and generalizing to other populations and research studies.

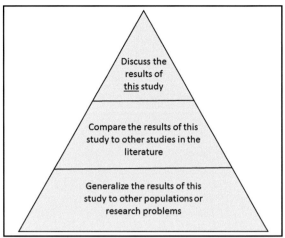

Discuss the results of <u>this</u> study

Compare the results of this study to other studies in the literature

Generalize the results of this study to other populations or research problems

them in a manner according to the science, from most to least important, or in a compare-and-contrast format. The organizational structure of the Discussion section should match the logic to form a solid, cohesive argument.

Some authors suggest that the Discussion section is written as a pyramid (Figure 2-1), which starts by specifically answering the study's research questions and finishes with generalizing the results to other populations and research studies.[3] A shell of the outline might look like this:

1. Interpret the results of this study
2. Compare the results to references and previous research
3. Generalize results
4. Acknowledge study limitations
5. Conclusion

Exercise 5

Review your list of brainstorming ideas and outline of the introduction. Which ideas are suitable for the Discussion section? Write out the outline for the discussion while noting any missing pieces.

Outlines for Book Chapters and Creative Works

Book chapters and creative works require a slightly different outlining technique. These types of manuscripts are not usually linear thought processes like journal articles, where one might go from point A to F by A – B – C – D – E – F. Book chapters and creative works have much more flexibility and can be rather fun to write once you get the hang of it. As long as an author's manuscript makes sense to the reader, it is just fine to take a different path from point A to F (A – B – D – E – B – E – C – F). The text needs to be logically organized, but there are many more options with book chapters and creative works, such as posters and oral/slide presentations. Because there are so many options with creative works, it is extremely important to organize one's thoughts prior to writing.

Traditional outlining like that used for research manuscripts works for some authors, but others insist on using a technique called *mind mapping*.[4] Mind mapping (Figure 2-2) a manuscript is similar to a map as the purpose statement is the center of the map (downtown) and main ideas radiate out from the center like neighborhoods around downtown. There can be many subideas represented under each main idea. After all ideas are placed on the map, lines or arrows are drawn between the ideas to connect them in a logical manner. These lines connecting ideas start looking like roads from downtown to the neighborhoods and from one neighborhood to another. Mind

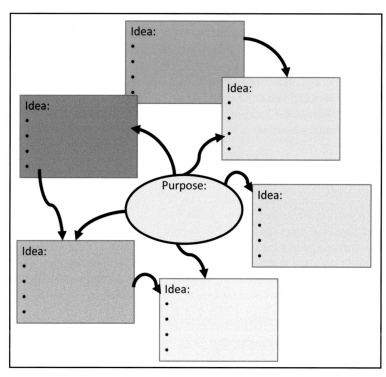

Figure 2-2. Example of mind mapping technique. Notice that all ideas relate to the purpose and some of the statements connect with others.

maps for longer works, such as books, could look like several cities (chapters) and joined by over-lapping ideas that will be covered in multiple chapters.

To get started with mind mapping, writers need to gather their supplies just like for a normal outline. Since mind mapping is more of a drawing tool, the following options are preferred by authors for this technique:

- Multiple sheets of paper and several colors of pens
- White board and colored markers
- Sticky notes
- Web-based apps (search the internet for mind mapping tools)
- Poster board and colored markers
- Butcher/Kraft paper and colored markers

Next, many authors will brainstorm ideas on a separate sheet of paper. Ideas do not have to be only words; feel free to use images and colors to help visualize the ideas. Once all the ideas are fleshed out and on paper (or other medium), all the ideas are organized and placed on the mind map. White boards and sticky notes are especially suited for the mind mapping technique.

Case Study

All of this seems like a lot of work and will take time to produce a quality outline. Could this time be better utilized writing? No, since a quality outline will keep manuscript writers on track and help prevent writer's block and off-topic writing. Off-topic writing is a huge issue when a manuscript (or book chapter) is written in small chunks of time. After each break due to work, family, travel, errands, etc; authors have to come back and find their place and start writing again. With an outline, there is less time wasted backtracking, allowing the author to immediately jump to the next point or where they left off before a break. If one is able to dedicate a couple hours a day to a writing project and write **every day**, then off-topic writing may not be an issue, but most authors do not have the time in their busy lives to schedule that type of time block for writing.

Consider the case of Georgina Campbell, who became famous for writing an entire book on her BlackBerry in 2012. She was a chef at the time and started writing on her BlackBerry because that is the one device that she always had with her. She wrote in small chunks of time whenever she had a few minutes. Her book *The Kickdown Girls* ended up being over 55,000 words and 202 pages! She was able to achieve this because she had prepared a strong outline and was just filling in the blanks when she had a few minutes to write.

Conclusion

Creating an outline prior to writing a manuscript or creative work is a must-do task and saves time and effort in the project timeline. Start the process by writing the purpose statement and then brainstorm ideas for the work. Organize the ideas according to topic or other natural group. Then drop the ideas into the fairly standard research manuscript format or, if the work is creative, organize to allow text to flow from one idea to the next. Writing with an outline saves time by preventing writing off-topic and often eliminates writer's block.

References

1. O'Connor DP, Laughlin MS, Woods GW. Factors related to additional knee injuries after anterior cruciate ligament injury. *Arthroscopy*. 2005;21(4):431-438. doi:10.1016/j.arthro.2004.12.004.
2. Morris BJ, Haigler RE, Laughlin MS, Elkousy HA, Gartsman GM, Edwards TB. Workers' compensation claims and outcomes after reverse shoulder arthroplasty. *J Shoulder Elb Surg*. 2014;Oct:1-7. doi:10.1016/j.jse.2014.07.009.
3. Hofmann AH. *Scientific Writing and Communication: Papers, Proposals and Presentations*. New York, NY: Oxford University Press; 2010:290-299.
4. Buzan T, Buzan B. *The Mind Map Book: How to Use Radiant Thinking to Maximize Your Brain's Untapped Potential*. New York, NY: Penguin Books USA Inc; 1996.

Bibliography

Annesley TM. The discussion section: your closing argument. *Clin Chem*. 2010;56(11):1671-1674. doi:10.1373/clinchem.2010.155358.

Foster A. *Writing a Book a Week: How to Write Quick Books Under the Self-Publishing Model*. Amazon Digital Services LLC; 2016.

Hofmann AH. *Scientific Writing and Communication: Papers, Proposals and Presentations*. New York, NY: Oxford University Press; 2010.

Silvia PJ. *How to Write a Lot*. Washington, DC: American Psychological Association; 2007.

Zeiger M. *Essentials of Writing Biomedical Research Papers*. 2nd ed. New York, NY: McGraw Hill; 2000.

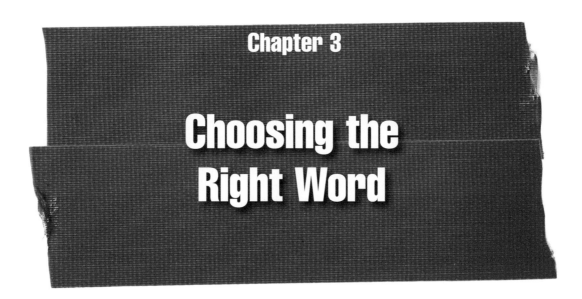

Chapter 3

Choosing the Right Word

Melissa Long, EdD, LAT, ATC, PES, LMT, CMT

Health care professionals communicate with a myriad of people. On any given day they can interact verbally with students, patients, doctors, parents, coaches, other health care professionals, and even insurance personnel. A special communication skill set can be required to effectively convey a message among all of these wide-ranging personalities, education levels, and levels of medical training. For example, it is important that health care professionals be able to adapt their communication tone and content to ensure that it can be understood by the patient yet also be able to effectively detail the intricacies of a diagnosis in order to coordinate appropriately with the therapy team. Likewise, all parties involved in a conversation must be able to understand the dialogue. However, oral communication can often include casual conversation and slang terminology that is not permissible in professional writing.

In addition to engaging in various levels of verbal communication, health care professionals must also be adept at clinical writing. Writing SOAP (subjective, objective, assessment, and plan) notes, progress notes, and home care plans are tasks performed regularly that can become somewhat routine for the health professional. However, clinic-based writing is different than technical or professional writing as it typically consists of short statements and brief comments regarding a patient's condition. Often times, clinical writing can be turned into professional or technical writing by simply completing sentences, fleshing out background information, or in some cases by simply choosing the right word. This chapter will concentrate on how manuscript writers can choose the right word in order to improve their technical and professional writing.

Conversation to Paper

In everyday speech, many words are often used to set a scene or describe a particular situation. Think about how an athlete might describe his or her mechanism of injury—it is most often very choppy (ie, noncomplete sentences), has poor flow from start to finish, and will likely include

Knoblauch M. *Professional Writing in Kinesiology and Sports Medicine* (pp 23-32).
© 2019 Taylor & Francis Group.

movements from the athlete to emphasize particular points. For example, if a football player sustained an injury, he might describe it as the following:

> I was running on 3rd and 10. I cut right and a defender was coming after me. I tried to juke left but got blindsided by another guy. He wrapped me up top but the other guy caught up and grabbed my legs. As I was falling I think the second guy hit the outside of my knee but I'm not really sure. It kind of bent in and I hit the ground. When they got off me I realized that my right knee hurt really bad. Kind of bent in a little bit but not too far. I was able to stand up and walk but it felt kind of wobbly or like it wasn't really strong on the inside. So I walked off the field. I tried to play a few more plays but I just couldn't do it. So I found my athletic trainer and he took a look at it.

While this description is great and sets the scene well, it would not be used in professional writing. The professionally written version of this paragraph should be much more concise by eliminating extraneous information as follows:

> The athlete was tackled, during which he sustained valgus blunt trauma to the right knee while weight-bearing. The athlete was able to walk off of the field but was unable to continue playing.

As the above example illustrates, quality professional writing requires very few words. This "less is more" ideology is a major tenet of professional writing in that an author should strive to get his or her point across in his or her writing in as few words as possible. However, to condense the information properly, the chosen words must be very succinct in nature.

To write successfully in a professional style, manuscript authors must use the correct words to convey their ideas properly yet concisely. This can be challenging, especially given the freedom most people employ in daily casual conversation compared to the rather strict constraints of professional writing. To illustrate this, the following are some examples from actual student work that illustrate how a more appropriate word choice would be beneficial. As outlined, alternative words can be used that convey the same thought but do not require the same amount of text.

Get some more = gain, increase

When the patient gets some more range of motion, he can return to work.

When the patient gains range of motion, he can return to work.

Going all the way = dating

He reported pain going all the way back to high school.

He reported pain dating back to high school.

Been able to go from = progressed

The patient had been able to go from 45 degrees to 60 degrees of range of motion.

The patient progressed from 45 degrees to 60 degrees of range of motion.

Had undergone = underwent

She had undergone 3 surgeries.

She underwent 3 surgeries.

Took the athlete through = completed

The physical therapist took the athlete through a full evaluation.

The physical therapist completed a full evaluation.

Being Clear and Concise

Professional and technical writing should be short, clear, and succinct. There is no need to add fillers or "fluff" to make the writing more interesting. Professional writing should use as few words as possible and the simplest language possible. Strunk and White[1] conveyed this idea well:

> Vigorous writing is concise. A sentence should contain no unnecessary words, a paragraph no unnecessary sentences, for the same reason that a drawing should have no unnecessary lines and a machine no unnecessary parts. This requires not that the writer make all his sentences short, or that he avoid all detail and treat his subjects only an outline, but that every word tell.

Prepositional Phrases

The simplest way to ensure one's writing is simple and clear is to avoid excessive use of prepositions and qualifiers. Prepositions such as *of, for, with, under, because,* and *by* can cause writing to become cluttered and hard to understand.[2] It is recommended that only 1 preposition be used for every 10 to 15 words in a sentence.[3] If an excessive number of prepositions occur in a sentence, replace some prepositions with noun strings, adverbs, verbs, or possessives.[4] Roberts[2(p115)] provided some examples of prepositional phrases and words to use in place of them.

During the course of = during

During the course of his treatment, the patient gained 25 pounds.

During his treatment, the patient gained 25 pounds.

In order to = to

In order to examine his foot, the physical therapist removed the shoe.

To examine his foot, the physical therapist removed the shoe.

Give consideration to = consider

The doctor must give consideration to the patient's work environment.

The doctor must consider the patient's work environment.

Qualifiers

Qualifiers such as *kind of, too, a little, very,* and *sort of* can cause writing to lose its strength persuasiveness.[2] Although these words are used often in verbal communication to qualify situations, they do not need to be included in professional writing. Qualifiers should be removed from writing whenever possible. If a knee is "a little" swollen or "very" swollen, it is still swollen. If the author feels it is necessary to include a qualifier, then it is best to do so with a quantitative measure such as girth measurements or pain scale rankings. Examples of unnecessary qualifiers are shown in the following.

A little

The patient's knee was a little swollen.

The patient's knee was swollen.

Kind of

The athlete was kind of upset about his injury.

The athlete was upset about his injury.

Quite

There was quite a bit of rain during the game.

There was rain during the game.

Abbreviated Words

In daily conversation within a clinic, medical professionals use a variety of words that are shortened versions of the whole word. While this saves time in conversation, those words should be written out completely in professional writing. Some of these shortened words are used so often that it is difficult to identify them as abbreviated versions of the original words. The following are some examples.

Rehab = rehabilitation

The rehab was successful.

The rehabilitation was successful.

Scope = arthroscope

The doctor will scope her knee.

The doctor will perform arthroscopic surgery on her knee.

Staph = staphylococcus infection

He had a staph infection.

He had a staphylococcus infection.

Reps = repetitions

She completed 3 sets of 10 reps.

She completed 3 sets of 10 repetitions.

Acronyms

Acronyms are very common in the medical world. Almost every medical organization has an acronym. In professional writing, it is acceptable to use acronyms, but only after it has been identified within the writing and then spelled out.[5] Once an acronym is defined, it can be used throughout the writing without further identification. The *Chicago Manual of Style* suggests that acronyms should be warranted 5 or more times in order to be used in a manuscript.[3] If an acronym would be used less than 5 times, then the whole series of words should be written out every time.[3]

It is important to note that specific to acronyms, many journals suggest that the author not start a sentence with an acronym and should instead write out the words. However, this does in turn add potentially unnecessary words to the manuscript. In many cases, authors can avert the need to write out the acronym's phrase at the beginning of a sentence by simply adding the word "The" before the acronym at the beginning of the sentence.

When writing for scientific journals or publications within the health community, common abbreviations such as MRI, CT, or CPR are often not spelled out. However, Kilshaw et al suggests that even these simple acronyms be spelled out the first time to avoid confusion.[6] It is important for authors to keep their target audience in mind during the manuscript phase when considering the use of acronyms. If the target audience is not familiar with certain medical terminologies, it will likely benefit the reader for the author to spell out the acronym prior to including it within the writing.

> *The National Athletic Trainers' Association (NATA) publishes consensus statements to help guide athletic trainers' (ATs') practice. The NATA consensus statement on spine-injured athletes is helpful when writing Emergency Action Plans (EAPs).*

When deciding whether to use an abbreviation or to spell out the complete series of words that make up the abbreviation, consider space within the paper or publication as well as the audience. Abbreviations can be used to help save space in a manuscript in that using abbreviations can help avoid cumbersome repetition. However, if the audience would benefit from seeing the whole phrase spelled out every time to avoid confusion, then that option may be best.[7]

Writing Out Numerals

Numbers are used quite often in scientific professional writing. It is generally accepted to use numerals for any number 10 and over. The standards for writing numbers below 10 are dependent upon the formatting system followed. The American Medical Association (AMA) format recommends using a numeral (eg, 4, 7, etc) when its use occurs within a sentence, although "one" should always be spelled out, unless it refers to a unit of measurement (1 cm) or time (1 week). It is also acceptable to use a numeral for 1 if other numbers are used later in the sentence. The American Psychological Association (APA) recommends the use of words when writing numbers 1 through 9 (eg, four, seven, etc).

> *The patient completed 3 sets of 7 repetitions. (AMA)*

> *The patient completed three sets of 15 repetitions. (APA)*

Whenever possible, avoid beginning a sentence with a number.[7] If starting a sentence with a numeral over 10 is to be avoided, rearranging the sentence to place the number further down the sentence will alleviate this issue.[8,9] If an author prefers to start a sentence with a number, that numeral should be spelled out.

> *Ninety-seven patients were seen in the clinic on Monday.*

> *On Monday, 97 patients were seen in the clinic.*

The rule specific to spelling out numbers less than 10 does have a few caveats. For example, when referencing page numbers, sizes, or percentages in professional writing, it is generally acceptable to use numbers even if they are under 10.

> *See page 7 for further instructions.*

> *A size 3 finger splint was used.*

> *After implementing the new exercises, an increase of about 6% of range of motion was achieved.*

Including dates in paragraphs can be tricky. If writing a specific date, be sure to spell out the month and include a comma between the date and the year. It is not necessary to include a th, rd, nd, or st when writing professionally.[9]

> *On March 3, 2017 the patient was admitted to the hospital.*

Generally, including specific dates in professional writing for publication is not necessary. For example, when writing a case report or other manuscript in which the patient's identity is blinded, it may behoove the author to write in a manner that avoids the use of specific dates. Be sure to check the *Author's Guide* of the publication for advanced guidance on this issue.

If the author wishes to include dates in his or her manuscript, the month and year are generally sufficient and it is not necessary to include a comma between said month and year.[9]

Roman numerals can be used in professional writing if they are a part of established terminology in the profession.[5,8] Examples of this would be stage IV cancer or grade II ankle sprain.

Contractions

Contractions should not be used in professional or scientific writing as they convey a colloquial level of writing that is not appropriate for professional writing.[10] Although the American Psychological Association manual does not directly ban the use of contractions, it does suggest that contractions reflect an informal tone.[7] Additionally, contractions can be confusing to people whose first language is not English. Contractions can be avoided by simply spelling out the words that were combined to make the contraction.

Slang

Slang words are used so often in everyday speech that most people do not even realize they are using slang. Often, people think the word *slang* refers to words that are used by a certain group of people to describe something that is normally not associated with that entity.[9] For example, the word *sick* is often used by a younger generation to describe something that is found to be extremely nice or exciting. A teenager may say to his friend, "That shirt is sick," which actually means the teenager likes the shirt. In a health care setting, the "sick" obviously means illness.

While slang is used in everyday speech, it is not considered acceptable in professional writing. Not only can the meaning of the word change over time, its literal meaning could be confused with its slang meaning. The words cool, hot, and sick are perfect examples of why slang words should not be used in professional settings. Although most people understand the commonly associated meanings of these words, it is important that the slang term not be used in professional writing because it could lead to confusion. In a health care setting, cool means not warm, whereas in slang terms cool can be interpreted to range from interesting to exciting. Hot literally means "having a relatively high temperature,"[11] however, the slang version could mean nice or even stolen. The multiple means of these words could cause misunderstandings and therefore only the traditional meaning of the word should be used in professional writing.

Slang terminology also factors into anatomically correct terms when writing professionally. Many slang terms have been widely accepted for numerous body parts such as shin, thigh, butt, and, neck, however, only anatomically correct terms should be used both in the clinic and in professional writing. The following are some examples.

Shin = tibia

Thigh = quadriceps or femur

Butt = gluteus maximus

Neck = cervical

Commonly Misused Words

In addition to slang terms, many words that are used on an everyday basis in the clinical setting are often misused to some degree. The following is a short list of words that are used often but are not used in the right context. While the following examples are common in verbal language, they are considered too informal for academic writing.[12] Following each example is a sentence outlining a more professional word to use in place of the misused term.

A lot = multiple

He completed a lot of sets.

He completed multiple sets.

A = per

She was in the clinic 6 hours a day.

She was in the clinic 6 hours per day.

Through = via

She completed 7 repetitions through the dynamometer.

She completed 7 repetitions via the dynamometer.

The Word Because

Historically, students are taught not to start a sentence with the word *because*. If one listens closely to verbal speech, sentences that begin with the word because are often fragmented sentences. Therefore, in order to avoid sentence fragments in writing, it is not recommended as a word to use for starting a sentence. However, as an author's writing becomes more professional and technical, using the word because to start a sentence can be done when it meets certain requirements. For example, in a cause and effect relationship, it is acceptable to start a sentence with because as it identifies the "cause" component of the sentence. It is important to ensure that if the cause is presented first in the sentence, then the effect follows after a comma. For example:

The patient began weight-bearing exercises because he was 6 weeks' postoperative.

Or:

Because he was 6 weeks' postoperative, the patient began weight-bearing exercises.

The optometrist wrote a prescription for a tinted visor because it was required by the NCAA.

Or:

Because a prescription was required by the NCAA, the optometrist wrote one for a tinted visor.

Occasionally, lessons learned early in school are deeply embedded and difficult to change. If this is the case, then often times the word because can be replaced with other representative words such as *due to, as a result of, as such*, etc. The following is an example.

Because she was 5 months pregnant, the patient could not lay on her stomach.

Becomes:

Due to the fact that she was 5 months pregnant, the patient could not lay on her stomach.

Reviewing Work

Reviewing work before submission is essential. However, reviewing one's own work is difficult. It is useful to find an outside reviewer who can objectively evaluate writing. This may be a peer or a mentor but could also be a hired editor. If an objective reviewer cannot be found, then one can review his or her own work, but should do so only after the writing is set aside for a few days or weeks and then taken back out and read from start to finish. Taking a short hiatus between writing and reviewing can often give the author a new perspective of his or her work.

Conclusion

Choosing the correct word in professional writing can make one's writing more clear and concise. Professional writing is not an easy task, and no one excels at it on his or her first try. Rather, it is a learned process that becomes more proficient each time it is practiced. Keep in mind that the way a person orally communicates is not necessarily the way information should be communicated in professional writing. Writers should take care to avoid slang terms, and instead choose words that have a clear and concise meaning. In addition, qualifiers and prepositions should be deleted when possible, along with ensuring sentences are not fragmented and taking time to begin sentences with appropriate words. The more the author practices professional writing components, the easier it will become to write well professionally.

Examples

As seen, it can be difficult initially to choose the correct word. When reading one's own original sentence it can seem easy to read and likely makes sense. However, after reading the corrected version of the same sentence, it becomes quite obvious that a more concise version improves the sentence's technical writing aspect, allows for the conveyance of the same thought, and requires much less text.

The following is an example that will walk through how to eliminate extraneous text, in turn making the sentence more concise.

Original:

I think this study gives a lot of insight to what is going on with athletic directors' current behaviors.

"I think" is written in first person, which should never be used in professional writing. It also weakens the author's argument.

This study gives a lot of insight to what is going on with athletic directors' current behaviors.

"gives" can be replaced with "provides" in order to sound more professional.

"a lot of" is a qualifier that is not quantifiable. Therefore, it should not be used.

This study provides insight to what is going on with athletic directors' current behaviors.

"to what" is not defined and is poor grammar.

"is going on" is full of prepositions.

This study provides insight into athletic directors' current leadership behaviors.

"Current behaviors" is vague. Including the word leadership gives more definition to the argument.

Corrected:

This study provides insight into athletic directors' current leadership behaviors.

The following are a few more examples. Work through the original and decide what changes should be made and why before reviewing the corrected version.

Original:

A limitation of the study was the potential sample, it was limited by the accuracy of the database they were provided, so they potentially missed out on participants due to inaccurate email addresses.

Corrected:

The sample was limited by the possibility of improperly addressed email.

Original:

Medial epicondylitis needs to be seen as an injury with no set path to follow while the pain and or symptoms can be very controlled or flare up at any time.

Corrected:

Medial epicondylitis has no predetermined pain control method or rehabilitation due to its individualized symptoms.

Original:

After rehabilitation implemented by the athletic trainers was showing no improvement in the patient's pain levels, it was then an indicator to move forward with consulting an orthopedic specialist.

Corrected:

The athlete's pain levels did not improve after completing strengthening exercises; therefore, an orthopedic surgeon was consulted.

Original:

As long as the department is set up to take on this task, transformational leaders can have a positive impact on the department.

Corrected:

If the department is prepared to employ this task, transformational leaders can have a positive impact on the department.

Original:

While taking her conditioning fitness assessment the athlete experienced some quad pain.

Corrected:

While completing her conditioning fitness assessment the athlete experienced quadriceps femoris pain.

References

1. Strunk W, White EB. *The Elements of Style*. 3rd ed. New York, NY: Macmillian; 1979.
2. Roberts CM. *The Dissertation Journey: A Practical and Comprehensive Guide to Planning, Writing, and Defending Your Dissertation*. 2nd ed. Thousand Oaks, CA: Corwin Press; 2010.
3. *The Chicago Manual of Style*. 17th ed. Chicago, IL: University of Chicago Press; 2017. doi:10.7208/cmos17.
4. Panter M. Editing tip: avoiding preposition overuse. https://www.aje.com/en/arc/editing-tip-avoiding-preposition-overuse/. Accessed December 31, 2017.
5. AMA Manual of Style Committee. *AMA Manual of Style: A Guide for Authors and Editors*. 10th ed. Oxford University Press; 2007.
6. Kilshaw MJ, Rooker J, Harding IJ. The use and abuse of abbreviations in orthopaedic literature. *Annals of The Royal College of Surgeons of England*. 2010;92(3):250-252.
7. *Publication Manual of the American Psychological Association*. 6th ed. Washington, DC: American Psychological Association; 2010.
8. *Concise Rules of APA Style*. Washington, DC: American Psychological Association; 2015.
9. Booth WC, Colomb GG, Williams JM, Turabian KL. *A Manual for Writers of Research Papers, Theses, and Dissertations: Chicago Style for Students and Researchers*. Chicago, IL: The University of Chicago Press; 2013.
10. Sabin WA, Millar WK, Strashok GW, Gardner LC. *The Gregg Reference Manual*. Whitby, Ontario, Canada: McGraw-Hill Ryerson; 2014.
11. *Merriam-Webster's Collegiate Dictionary*. 10th ed. Springfield, MA: Merriam-Webster Inc; 1999.
12. English language and usage. Retrieved from https://english.stackexchange.com/questions/62009/difference-between-per-and-a

Chapter 4

Basic Sentence Structure

Jon Gray, EdD

To be an effective writer, one must understand sentence structure. Basic sentence structure is not necessarily the most enjoyable topic to study; however, applying sentence concepts appropriately is essential in professional writing.[1] The communication of basic sentence structure serves as a guide to answer common questions related to writing.[2] The information in this chapter may come across as somewhat simplistic, and that is partially by design. Writers can use this chapter as a guide to answer common questions related to their writing. In addition, this chapter discusses many terms related to sentence structure as well as some do's and don'ts of writing. Although the content of basic sentence structure is information that all authors have studied at some point in the past and use daily, the reality is that many may be seeing this information for the first time or are revisiting the topic after a substantial lapse in time. Therefore, the overall purpose of this chapter is to provide a framework of basic sentence structure by identifying basic sentence terminology and providing examples of these terms as well as the various types of sentences. In addition, common mistakes writers make as well as various qualities of good writers are discussed. It is important to keep in mind that it is impossible to cover all of the rules in the writing process in one chapter. Therefore, the focus of this chapter is on the "basics" of creating sentences and some of the major pitfalls and strengths of good writers.

Basic Sentence Terms

Before beginning a discussion of sentence types as well as the various purposes of different sentences, it would be best to revisit basic sentence terms for review purposes. In this section, we will operationally define these basic sentence terms as well as provide examples of each. The reader should keep in mind that this is not an inclusive list of terms but rather a starting point to effectively construct sentences and communicate thoughts.

Knoblauch M. *Professional Writing in Kinesiology and Sports Medicine* (pp 33-42).
© 2019 Taylor & Francis Group.

Nouns

Everyone remembers learning about nouns at some point, but after years outside of an English classroom it may be difficult to explain what they are. A noun is a part of speech that identifies a person, place, thing, or idea. Nouns are incredibly important in written language, but they are also easy to understand. Understanding how nouns function in sentences is the building block of understanding more advanced rules when writing.

Nouns identify people, places, things, and ideas. Nouns can be categorized as either common or proper. Common nouns name general people, places, things, and ideas, while proper nouns name specific people, places, things, and ideas.[3,4]

Examples of common nouns:

school

player

patient

supplement

professor

Examples of proper nouns:

University of Anywhere

Jordan Smith

Jane Doe

Dr. John Doe

Verbs

A verb is one of the main parts of a sentence or question. Every proper sentence must have a verb—a word or group of words that says something about the subject, indicating action, possession, or state of being. Whether mental, physical, or mechanical, verbs always express activity. Verbs constitute the root of the predicate, which, along with the subject, forms a sentence.[3,4]

Examples of verbs:

The student <u>is</u> responsible.

The athlete <u>threw</u> the ball.

The students <u>measured</u> the distance.

Verb Phrases

Writers need to understand the use of verb phrases to write professionally. Verb phrases help to make the text more informative and meaningful and they are essential in the writing process. Verb phrases take the verb one step further by comprising the verb, plus the complement, object, or adverb. So, a verb phrase is a group of words that consists of a main verb and all of its helping verbs. A verb phrase can be the predicate (ie, what the subject does) of a sentence or the clause of a sentence. Often, a helping verb is used in addition to the verb. A helping verb is a verb that comes before the main verb.[3,4] While writing professionally, a helping verb will add meaning to a sentence that cannot be expressed by the main verb.

Examples of verb phrases:

I <u>may</u> work out today.

I <u>must</u> work out today.

The athlete <u>is lifting</u> weights.

The athlete <u>had been resting</u>.

Subjects

Every sentence has a subject, which is a word or group of words that names or indicates a person or thing that tells what the sentence is about. A subject is probably the most basic unit in sentence construction. A subject is a noun, which is a person, place, thing, or idea. A subject tells us who or what the sentence is going to be about. Without a subject, writers cannot generate a true complete sentence. A subject has just one noun as the focus of the sentence. This means that only one noun does the action or connects to the verb of the sentence. However, keep in mind that a subject can include modifiers of the noun. Noun modifiers are used in professional writing to better describe the noun. When noun modifiers are used the subject will become a phrase, not just a word.[3,4]

Examples of subjects:

<u>We</u> like football.

The <u>student</u> is responsible.

Both <u>experience</u> and <u>education</u> are necessary.

<u>Everything</u> on the agenda has been discussed.

The tough <u>athlete</u> has a high pain tolerance.

The smart <u>student</u> is studying.

Predicates

The predicate in a sentence expresses what the subject of the sentence does. The predicate in a sentence always includes a verb. While writing professionally, it is acceptable to have a predicate that consists of just the verb, or the predicate can consist of the verb as well as the descriptive words that come along with it. A complete sentence must include a subject and a predicate, and a predicate can be just a verb by itself or a verb with an additional description.[3,4]

Examples of predicates:

He <u>is an experienced athlete</u>.

The professor <u>lives in town</u>.

The student <u>has been studying</u>.

He <u>will hit</u> the ball.

Prepositions

Writers use prepositions to relate items to each other. Specifically, prepositions are short words that indicate place, motion, cause, and time. Those that indicate place include *in, on, at, near, beside, along, among, over,* or *under.* Some prepositions that indicate motion are *from, toward, up, down, around, into,* or *onto.* Many prepositions show cause, such as *because of, for, with,* or *by.*

Examples of prepositions that indicate time include *since*, *to*, *past*, and *until*. English has more than 100 words that can be used as prepositions.[3,4]

Prepositional Phrases

The basic function of prepositions is to show how a noun relates to the rest of the sentence. That noun is called the "object of the preposition." For example, in the sentence "The physical education teacher is at the field," "at the field" is the prepositional phrase and "field" is the object of the preposition. A prepositional phrase is a group of words consisting of a preposition and its object plus any modifiers of the preposition or the subject.[3,4]

Examples of prepositional phrases:

The athletic trainer is <u>in the athletic training room</u>.

The physical education teacher is <u>at the field</u>.

The graduate student is <u>down the hall</u>.

The injured athlete is <u>on the table</u>.

Clause

A clause is a group of words that have a subject and a predicate and that are used as a part of a sentence. There are 2 kinds of clauses: main clauses, also called *independent* clauses, and subordinate clauses, also called *dependent* clauses. Like a prepositional phrase or a noun phrase, a clause is a group of related words; but unlike a phrase, a clause has a subject and verb. An independent clause, along with having a subject and verb, expresses a complete thought and can stand alone as a coherent sentence. In contrast, a subordinate or dependent clause does not express a complete thought and, therefore, is not a sentence. A subordinate clause standing alone is a common error known as a *sentence fragment*.[3,4]

A main clause contains a subject that lets the reader know what the sentence is about, as well as a verb that informs the readers what the subject is doing or will do. Since a main clause has a subject and a predicate, and contains enough information, it can stand alone as a sentence.

Example of a main clause:

<u>Physical therapy is a popular field of study</u>.

A subordinate clause has a subject and a predicate, but it cannot stand alone as a sentence. A subordinate clause cannot stand alone because it does not include enough necessary information to be a complete sentence. A subordinate clause must have a main clause attached to it. Often times, a subordinate clause uses words like *although*, *because*, *before*, or *after*.[4]

Example of a subordinate clause:

Physical therapy is a popular field of study <u>because of its high demand in the workforce</u>.

A Sentence

A sentence is a set of words that is a complete expression or thought. A sentence can take the form of a question, a statement, an expression, or a command. A sentence can consist of a clause or several clauses. When discussing sentences, it is important to distinguish between sentence structure and sentence purpose. The type of the sentence (structure) and the way or direction in which it is written (purpose) both contribute to the overall clarity of the sentence. In scientific writing, both of these sentence characteristics are vital, as they communicate a specific message to be delivered to the reader.

Types of Sentences

It is important to identify the 4 sentence structures or types of sentences. The 4 sentence types include: simple, compound, complex, and compound-complex.[5] In this section are the operational definitions and examples of the 4 sentence types and examples of each.

A simple sentence has only one main clause and no subordinate clauses.

Example of a simple sentence:

Exercise physiology is a popular field of study.

A compound sentence has 2 or more main clauses.

Example of a compound sentence:

Exercise physiology is a popular field of study, and more students are choosing this as their major.

A complex sentence has one main clause and one or more subordinate clauses.

Example of a complex sentence:

Although more classes have been added to the curriculum, I chose not to go into physical therapy.

A compound-complex sentence has more than one main clause and at least one subordinate clause.

Example of a compound-complex sentence:

Because of the popularity of sports medicine, classes have been added, and the curriculum is being scrutinized.

Purposes of Sentences

Just as there are 4 sentence types or structures, there are also 4 different purposes of sentences. When a writer understands the different purposes of sentences that make up the written language, then he or she can better compose words to express a variety of thoughts and emotions. Expressing thoughts and emotions is essential to scientific writing in order to best provide facts, provoke thought, or raise questions about future research. The 4 directional purposes of sentences are declarative, imperative, interrogative, and exclamatory,[5] from which there are 3 punctuation marks with which to end a sentence; a period, a question mark, and an exclamation point. The punctuation that ends the sentence and the purpose of the sentence are directly related. The following are the definitions and examples of the 4 purposes of a sentence:

A declarative sentence simply makes a statement or expresses an opinion. Therefore, it makes a declaration and ends with a period.

Example of a declarative sentence:

I'm coming to class tonight.

An imperative sentence gives a command or makes a request. It usually ends with a period but can, under certain circumstances, end with an exclamation point.

Example of an imperative sentence:

You're coming to class tonight.

An interrogative sentence asks a question. This type of sentence often begins with who, what, where, when, why, how, or do, and typically ends with a question mark.

Example of an interrogative sentence:

Who is coming to class tonight?

An exclamatory sentence is a sentence that expresses great emotion such as excitement, surprise, happiness and anger, and ends with an exclamation point.

Example of an exclamatory sentence:

I will be coming to class tonight!

It is important to note that most scientific writing is the communication of facts. Therefore, professional writers most often use declarative sentences in their writing. When authors write declaratively, they disseminate relevant information about a topic or issue based on available literature. Scientific writers, editors, and publishers may use the other 3 types of sentences (imperative, interrogative, exclamatory) from time to time, however, declarative writing is the standard.

Good Writing

Good writing makes reading easy. Good writing anticipates reader questions and serves to answer those questions before the reader asks. It is always important to keep in mind that words matter. In addition to what is written, the style it is written in, or how something is said, quality writing is a unique gift in communicating with the reader. In this section, 3 qualities of good writing are outlined.

Good Writing Is Consistent

To be a consistent writer, focus on the overall message. While writing, authors must continuously ask themselves, "Does this word or sentence assist the reader in understanding the main idea or concept I am communicating?" Too often, writers create thoughts or ideas that take readers away from the main objectives or themes of the piece they are writing. If a sentence does not help the reader understand the main concept, then do not use it.[5]

In addition, consistent writers develop the same pattern with word choice and punctuation. Stay consistent with names and terminology while writing. To illustrate, do not use Dr. Gray, Mr. Gray, Professor Gray, and Jon interchangeably within the same body of work. Doing so will require the reader to think about to whom the author is exactly referring. The same can be said about terminology; do not switch between scientific and common terms in writing.

Punctuation must also be consistent. As mentioned in the following "Common Sentence Mistakes" section, punctuation is often misused throughout a document, and consequently the message that the writer is trying to communicate is lost. This loss of the message is often associated with comma use. Often times the use of a comma is left up to the choice of the writer. In other words, it may be acceptable to include or leave out a comma while writing professionally. In manuscript writing, the author must use the comma consistently throughout the document. For example, when using the word *too*, it is not necessary to use a comma. However, if placing a comma before the word too, such as in the sentence "He threw the ball, too" then it is important to remain consistent and use the comma before "too" throughout the text.

Good Writing Is Simple

Good writers stubbornly and persistently think about their writing from the reader's perspective. Good writing is like good officiating; just as a good official or umpire should not get in the way of the flow of a game, good sentence development should not hinder or slow the momentum of the reading process.[5]

To keep writing simple, first think about the main idea that is to be communicated to the reader, and then write that idea as simply as possible. This can be tricky because ideas can often be complex and detailed; however, the outlining of ideas does not have to be complex or detailed.

In order to keep one's writing simple, it may be necessary to break down complex concepts into steps or categories. For example, when writing about a beneficial workout routine, write about the workout from conception to the end instead of writing about all aspects of the workout at once. Therefore, start by discussing the warm-up, then stretching, then the main work out, cool-down, then stretching again. The reader can then visualize the workout as well as the flow of the workout.

Good Writing Is Clear

Writing is a conversation between the writer and the reader. Clarity in writing helps readers understand concepts and important details. When communicating orally, a presenter can modify the tone of his or her voice or use hand gestures. But a writer must rely on other tools. One tool a writer can use to increase clarity is to use bold and/or italics to add significance to his or her writing. However, be careful to not overuse bold and italics. A general rule to consider is, if everything has to be emphasized when writing then emphasize nothing. Secondly, another tool to increase clarity is to use examples. Examples can make a general concept specific or an abstract idea concrete. Furthermore, examples should be specific to the intended audience and should be short, concise, and simplistic. Lastly, promote clarity by writing specifically for the intended audience. When writing, keep in mind the audience's characteristics and write accordingly. Obviously, writing should be different for a class of fifth graders than writing for post-doctorate scholars. In addition, writers should take into account the audience's areas of interests and expertise. For example, using specific medical terminology while writing for a group of medical professionals is both appropriate and expected, whereas using the same medical terminology for a group of cancer patients requires further explanation or should not be used.

Common Sentence Mistakes in Professional Writing

Mistakes in the writing process are inevitable, even for the most accomplished writer. However, a writer can limit these mistakes simply by recognizing common mistakes while writing. This section discusses some of the more common writing mistakes made in sentence writing. Again, writers must keep in mind that this is not an all-inclusive list but rather an example of common errors.

Comma

The purpose of the comma is to have a slight pause or hesitation in a sentence. If uncertain of whether or not to use a comma in a given sentence, read the sentence aloud and see if it sounds better with or without a pause, and then add or omit the comma. Additionally, it may be helpful to use text-to-voice programs (eg, Microsoft Word) that will verbalize the text. Too often a comma is used when the sentence will read better without a pause. However, if a comma is not used with 2 or more independent clauses (ie, complete sentences), a run-on sentence will result. Run-on sentences can often be fixed by utilizing a comma or semicolon along with a coordinating conjunction like "and" or "but" between the 2 clauses, or in some cases separating the clauses into 2 independent sentences. It should be noted that there are many rules associated with commas, and discussing every rule will probably cause more confusion than clarity. Here are a few simple examples of comma usage.

Examples of correct use of a comma:

Finally, I lifted weights.

While lifting weights, I listened to hip hop, a type of music.

Examples of incorrect use of a comma:

John, and Mark lifted weights.

John and Mark have a new workout routine, because they lost their old one.

Semicolon

Another common mistake is the misuse of the semicolon. A semicolon is both a comma and a period. Its purpose is to serve as a hard pause or as a period. The writer may want to use a semicolon as a hard pause to separate 2 independent clauses with a conjunction. Often times a writer will use a semicolon to bring together independent statements more closely than a period allows.

Examples of correct and incorrect semicolon usage:

The athletic trainer taped my ankle today; he was very fast.

Not

The athletic trainer taped my ankle today. He was very fast.

Also:

The pitcher has a nasty curve ball; he loves to throw it during practice.

Not

The pitcher has a nasty curve ball; and he loves to throw it during practice.

Reader-Friendly Writing

Writers often worry about the flow of their writing, such as whether their writing does not make sense or if a sentence does not fit its intended purpose. Worrying about one's writing can be good, as it can serve to produce a better overall product. There are many ways in which writing does not flow well or make sense to readers. This section explores 2 areas—creating stand-alone sentences and sentence transitioning—that can assist writers to make reading easier as well as increase the "flow" of their writing.

Stand-Alone Sentences

Writers and readers should be able to take a sentence out of a paper, read it, and not be left with any questions as to the intent or content of the sentence. Furthermore, readers should not be left wondering to what any words in that sentence may be referring. One way to assist writers with writing stand-alone sentences is by using clear and concise wording. Clear and concise wording also creates flow.[6] Take this sentence:

Clinical experiences, which means hands-on experiences out in the field, can help a student become more competent in the field, which may help a student get recognized for his or her good work and receive a job.

Trying to include "everything" that the writer is wanting to discuss creates quite a long sentence. All of the phrases or ideas are stacked on top of the other, and the reader must maneuver too much through the sentence to fully understand the intent of the sentence. Even if broken into multiple sentences, the thoughts conveyed in poorly designed sentences can be problematic. For example:

> *Clinical experiences can help a student become more competent. They can help them get recognized for his or her good work and receive a job.*

The use of "they" and "them" in the second sentence is somewhat confusing as to what subject it is referring. Does "they" refer to clinical experiences or students? As written, the sentence cannot be understood without referring back to the previous sentence, in turn requiring more effort on the part of the reader in order to understand the author's intent (think back to the basketball officiating reference discussed earlier). As discussed previously, each sentence should stand alone and not leave any question as to the intent or content of the sentence. Now, consider the following sentence:

> *Clinical experiences help students become competent in the field, which can ultimately result in recognition or promotion for those students.*

This sentence has the same meaning as the previous sentence but is more concise and easier to follow. Furthermore, it does not leave the reader with any unreferenced subjects that require explanation based on prior sentences. Using concise wording is like taking a direct route while traveling in a car. Rather than taking the reader through the ups and downs and turns of all the back roads, the writer should take the reader directly to the main idea.

Transitions

Transitions can mean transitioning from one thought or idea to another or it can mean that the sentence fits into the context that is written. Transitioning from one sentence to another creates flow to writing and assists the reader's comprehension of the main idea of the sentence or paragraph.[6] Each sentence should both follow the direction of the preceding sentence as well as lead into the next sentence. To aid writers in maintaining proper sentence flow, transitional words and/or phrases can be used in navigating from one sentence to the next. Some of the commonly used transitional words and/or phrases include *for example, for instance, as a result, therefore,* and *specifically.* To illustrate, let us take a look at 3 sentences that build on one another using transition words:

> *While the research experiment was conducted at a university in Utah, researchers did not find any evidence that altitude was considered to be a factor.*

> *In addition, another experiment in Texas produced similar results, where participants were only 20 feet above sea level.*

> *Therefore, the researchers concluded that altitude did not play a factor in the results.*

Conclusion

As mentioned throughout the chapter, it is impossible to cover all of the terminology, rules, and exceptions in the writing process in one chapter. Hopefully, what has been covered in this chapter can serve as a guide for improving one's writing, and the information presented should serve as a viable refresher for manuscript writers.

Writing is a continuous process of revising and editing, and forming quality sentences is one of the key steps in the writing process. As discussed, writing starts with prewriting and continues until the last draft best fits the writer's intended purpose. An individual's writing will miss its intended purpose if basic sentence terms and structures are not followed. Therefore, it is essential that writers scrutinize their writing style for proper grammar usage and concepts. Writing is similar to everything else—the more experience attained, the better one will become.

References

1. Knight KL, Ingersoll D. Optimizing scholarly communication: 30 tips for writing clearly. *J Athl Train.* 1996;31(3):209-213.
2. Linte CA. Tips on scientific writing and manuscript preparation. *IEEE Pulse.* 2014;Nov/Dec:58-60.
3. Faulkner CW. *Writing Good Sentences: A Functional Approach to Sentence Structure Grammar, and Punctuation.* New York, NY: Charles Scriber's Sons; 1957.
4. *Macmillan English.* New York, NY: Scribner Educational Publishers; 1986.
5. Dexter P. Tips for scholarly writing in nursing. *J Prof Nurs.* 2000;16(1):6-12.
6. Clark RP. *Writing Tools: 50 Essential Strategies for Every Writer.* Boston, MA: Little Brown & Company; 2008.

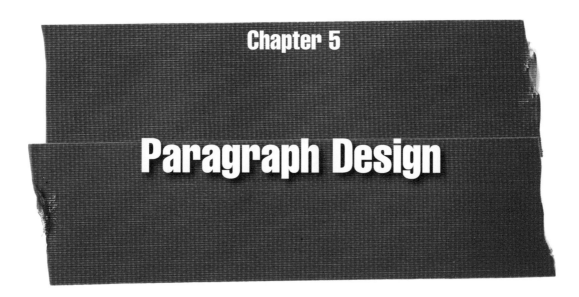

Chapter 5

Paragraph Design

Mitzi S. Laughlin, PhD, LAT, ATC

Paragraphs are one of several key pieces that come together to form a great paper. The right words form the right sentence. The right sentences build a strong paragraph. The right paragraph completes the right section. And the right sections solidify the work into a great paper. So the right words, sentences, paragraphs, and sections are needed for a great paper (Figure 5-1). The right words and sentence structure were covered in the previous chapters; thus, this chapter will focus on building strong paragraphs.

A paragraph can be any collection of sentences, but a strong paragraph has many carefully constructed elements within the collection of sentences. To write a strong paragraph, an author must be able to present the topic in a clear, organized manner to the reader.

One Paragraph, One Idea

The first rule of a strong paragraph is that one paragraph includes one—and only one—idea or concept. Paragraphs with more than one idea or concept are more difficult for a reader to understand. If there is more than one idea in a paragraph, split the paragraph into several paragraphs until there is only one idea included in each paragraph.

Exercise 1

Read the following paragraph and determine if multiple ideas are incorporated:

The risk of additional injuries to the knee menisci and articular cartilage increases over time after anterior cruciate ligament (ACL) injury. Meniscus tears and articular cartilage lesions in an ACL-deficient knee can contribute to the development of arthrosis and other disabling knee conditions. Women have a higher incidence rate of ACL injury than men. Long delays between ACL injury and ACL reconstruction have been shown to be associated with increased occurrence rates of meniscus and articular cartilage injuries. Meniscus injuries associated with an ACL injury are less frequent when ACL reconstruction is performed within 4 to 6 weeks of

Knoblauch M. *Professional Writing in Kinesiology and Sports Medicine* (pp 43-51).
© 2019 Taylor & Francis Group.

Figure 5-1. Key components of a great paper.

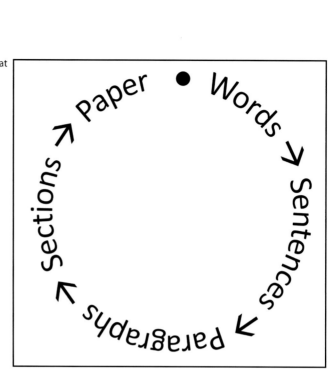

injury, as opposed to more than 6 months after ACL injury. The occurrence rate of articular cartilage lesions associated with an ACL injury has also been reported to be lower in the acute phase of injury (0% to 19%) than in the chronic phase (48% to 66%). Persons who participate in vigorous physical activities have been shown to be more disabled by an ACL injury than are patients who are relatively sedentary.[1]

Although the general topic of the paragraph is additional knee injuries following ACL injury, there are 2 sentences that do not fit within this paragraph:

1. Women have a higher incidence rate of ACL injury than men.
2. Persons who participate in vigorous physical activities have been shown to be more disabled by an ACL injury than are patients who are relatively sedentary.

These 2 sentences are structurally sound and factually correct, but do not fit within this paragraph that describes additional knee injuries following ACL injury. Consequently, both sentences need to be removed from this paragraph and saved for a paragraph with a different focus. For example, the sentence about women having a higher incidence rate of ACL injuries would be a good supporting sentence for a paragraph describing the risk factors of ACL injuries.

Paragraph Structure

Paragraphs for scientific manuscripts are fairly straightforward and usually follow a pattern that can be adapted to most research questions. An effective paragraph has a strong topic sentence that contains the main idea or concept presented in the paragraph. Sometimes this sentence is called an *overview* or *introductory* sentence but the function is the same—introduce the idea or concept of the paragraph and frame the message of the paragraph. Usually this sentence is the first sentence of the paragraph, but it could be anywhere in the paragraph. A good topic sentence introduces the new idea and also references the idea from the previous paragraph. Often this topic sentence is of a general nature while the subsequent sentences provide more details to support the topic sentence. A short and simple topic sentence can be a powerful statement that leads the reader into the details of the paragraph.

As noted, the middle sentences of a paragraph provide more details supporting the topic sentence. The order of the middle sentences is based on logic of the particular topic. For example, the middle sentences can be presented chronologically, most severe to least severe, or compare and contrast. Any of these methods are fine but need to be matched to the particular topic of the paragraph. The middle sentences provide the most details to the reader by giving facts and examples while often referencing the literature. When writing these middle sentences, writers should refer back to the topic sentence frequently and make sure the information included in the middle sentences remains relevant to the topic sentence. If it is not relevant, move the sentence to another paragraph or delete. Overall, these middle sentences provide the rationale for the topic sentence and give the details supporting the topic.

The final sentence in a paragraph is a concluding sentence. This sentence brings the paragraph to a logical conclusion and possibly leads into the next paragraph. Many authors restate the topic sentence or summarize the findings of the paragraph for the concluding sentence. Depending on the section, the concluding sentence may be a special format. For example, the last sentence of the introduction is usually reserved for the purpose of the paper statement. Most paragraphs contain a concluding sentence but not all. For long or complex paragraphs, consider a concluding sentence to help the reader summarize the main idea of the paragraph.

Exercise 2

The following sentences are taken from the published article *Preoperative Opioid Use and Outcomes After Reverse Shoulder Arthroplasty.*[2] Rearrange the sentences into a strong paragraph.

1. Opioid medications are being used more commonly as a nonoperative modality to treat chronic musculoskeletal conditions, including osteoarthritis-associated pain.

2. The use of opioid medications may lead to tolerance, hyperalgesia, and worse treatment outcomes.

3. CTA is a chronic condition, and most patients ultimately require operative treatment to improve function and provide pain relief; however, an initial trial of nonoperative treatment is typically warranted, including activity modification, anti-inflammatory medications, oral analgesics, corticosteroid injections, and gentle range of motion exercises.

4. Reverse shoulder arthroplasty (RSA) was originally designed for the treatment of rotator cuff tear arthropathy (CTA), and CTA remains the most common indication for RSA.

Answer: 4 – 3 – 1 – 2

Building Strong Paragraphs

A strong paragraph is one unit of writing and should be able to stand on its own. At a minimum, this requires a good paragraph structure—introductory sentence, supporting sentence(s), and then a concluding sentence. Many other components help create a strong paragraph and are discussed in the next several sections. Depending on factors such as the topic, writing style, or section of the manuscript, it is possible that one, all, or none of the components will be used in a paragraph (Sidebar 5-1).

Logical Order

A paragraph that stands on its own demonstrates a logical order or argument with no missing pieces. For example, if an introductory sentence describes risk factors for ACL injuries and lists age, gender, and sport played, then the supporting sentences need to address age, gender, and sport played. If an author does not mention the sport played in the supporting sentences, then there

Sidebar 5-1

When should I start a new paragraph?
- To introduce a new topic or idea
- To contrast opinions or arguments about a topic
- To give the readers a break
- Before you fill the entire page

would be a missing piece to the logical order of the paragraph. Similarly, if an author includes playing surface or shoe type as risk factors in the supporting sentences, then the paragraph is not adhering to a logical argument. If the author wants to discuss multiple risk factors of ACL injuries in a paragraph and there are too many to list in the introductory sentence, then the author can write an open-ended introductory sentence that allows discussing multiple risk factors as needed.

Another facet to logical order is the actual order of the supporting statements. There are many ways to order the statements depending on the particular research topic:
- Chronological order
- Most to least important
- Follow a process—Steps 1, 2, 3, and 4
- Cause and effect
- Define and then give examples
- Compare and contrast

Length

Depending on the topic, a paragraph may be any length, from a couple of sentences to something much, much longer. The shortest paragraph could be a single word like "Go" but that will rarely be appropriate in scientific writing. One of the longest sentences in the English language is credited to William Faulkner from *Absalom, Absalom!* and is a staggering 1,288 words. But authors beware—long sentences and long paragraphs are difficult on the readers. Text needs to be broken up into paragraphs for easier understanding and to develop a logical argument. Too long of a paragraph and the reader gets lost and is not able to follow the author's logic. Another reason to break up a long chunk of text is just to give the reader a break. Long passages are taxing to the eye and sometimes look daunting and the reader gets lost and has to start over, or worse, skips to the next article. So, authors should help their readers out and choose their paragraph length wisely. In scientific writing, a paragraph is usually 4 to 8 sentences but should be on the lower end if each of the sentences are long and complex. A manuscript writer should remember to be gentle on readers and be organized with his or her paragraphs (Sidebar 5-2).

References—But Not Too Many

When an author develops a paragraph, many of the support statements will use ideas from other articles and therefore need to be referenced. Be diligent in referencing to avoid plagiarism (see Chapters 8 and 14), but there is a fine line between referencing appropriately and including too many references. An author should select the most relevant articles to reference. Many times these are original articles that discuss the topic or issue. Do not fall into the trap of referencing only the articles that can be found easily or that another paper referenced. Rather, authors should go back and find the original articles to cite.

Another strategy for appropriately referencing is to cite the most important, best written, or the most recent paper on the topic. Avoid overreferencing common statements where there could be literally thousands of references. For example, the statement "Women have a higher incidence rate of ACL injury than men" has been discussed in thousands of journal articles and books. An author does not need to find every reference. Pick 1, 2, or maybe 3 and be done with it. As a general guideline, the original article to mention the idea is always good to reference and then possibly a newer article. Other authors choose a review article that covers many of the articles that are covered in the new manuscript.

Consistent Topic Order

When writing a strong paragraph, a writer needs to be consistent with the order of topics. If the introductory sentence mentions different treatment modalities and lists ice, heat, muscle stimulation, ultrasound, and stretching, then the supporting sentences need to be in the same order. Keeping the same order of topics helps the reader follow along and understand the paragraph easier. If the order is not the same in the introduction and support sentences, change one or the other. It does not matter which one is changed but just be consistent.

Consistent Terminology

The terminology used in sports medicine can be technical and sometimes confusing to the average reader. Many conditions or treatments have several commonly used names, for example, total knee arthroplasty, total knee, knee replacement, knee replacement surgery, and knee joint replacement. Which one does an author use in a manuscript? It depends on the intended audience. If the article is aimed at professionals, then total knee arthroplasty is the appropriate terminology. But if the article is focused on educating patients about their upcoming surgery, then one of the other terms may be more familiar to a particular patient. To avoid confusion, an author may state something like, "Your doctor has recommended a knee replacement, also commonly known as [and list all the terms]." The idea is to be consistent with the terminology as paragraphs and articles written with consistent terminology are easier on the reader.

Minimal Use of Technical Jargon

All professions seem to speak in their own language. Reading any professional literature requires a certain amount of inside knowledge and technical jargon, but authors should try to minimize the use. Some of the worst examples of technical jargon come from NASA, but the medical profession has its share also. Medical terms describing range of motion can be confusing to the layperson so in patient education articles an author should use "bend and straighten your knee" rather than knee flexion and extension. Scientific articles written to educate other professionals usually have more jargon because peers understand the language. But remember, this jargon can make new professionals, students, and patients feel like outsiders as they might not understand the jargon. If in doubt, leave out the jargon and use terms everyone understands.

Exercise 3

The following sentence is written for a medical audience. Rewrite the sentence so it can be used in a patient education brochure.

We conducted a study to examine shoulder function scores, mobility, patient satisfaction, and complications at minimum 2-year follow-up in normal-weight, overweight, and obese patients who underwent shoulder surgery.[3]

Varied Sentence Structure

A strong paragraph will vary the sentence structure and style. Overuse of one sentence structure can become monotonous for both the reader and author. Mix long sentences with a few short sentences. Sentence type should also be varied as too many sentences starting with "The study … " becomes boring fast. An article will flow easier by mixing simple, compound, complex, and compound-complex sentences. Do not worry if there is difficulty in remembering the sentence types from English class, just realize that sentence structure should be varied. This can be accomplished by inserting a phrase at the beginning or end of the sentence or by changing a statement with a conjunction (and, but, or, so) into an independent or dependent clause. Overall, an author should avoid repetition of one type of sentence structure to help the article flow and add variety to the writing. For more help on sentence structure, refer to Chapter 4 of this book.

Transitions

A solid paragraph needs to have continuity with the paragraph before and after. Similarly, each sentence in a paragraph needs to have continuity with the ones before and after. So how does an author provide continuity within a work? Transitions. Transitions are so important, they should be an author's best friend.

Transition words and phrases indicate the relationship between sentences and paragraphs. Transitions ensure that the reader understands how each sentence is related to the others. Most transitional words occur at the beginning of the sentence and are separated with a comma (Sidebar 5-3).

Phrases can also be used as transitions between both sentences and paragraphs. Transitional phrases are simple propositional phrases that explain the logical relationship between ideas. "For example" is a frequently used transitional phrase when the author wants to give examples of the idea presented in the previous sentence. Other common transition phrases include:

- In addition to X
- As a result of Y
- In conclusion

Use transition words and phrases to make the logical relationship between ideas known to the reader, but do not overuse them. Sometimes repetitive word choices make the relationship clear and no transition is needed. Similar to sentence structure, vary the use of transition words and phrases to make reading and understanding the manuscript easier on the reader.

Repetition as Links

Another technique for smooth transitions from one sentence or paragraph to another is repeating key words. A writer can repeat a noun, pronoun, synonym, and verbs with similar meanings to link several sentences together to create an interconnected effect. This is a powerful technique. Read the following example and evaluate whether the bolded words help transition from one idea to another.

> *Reverse shoulder arthroplasty (RSA) was originally designed for the treatment of rotator* ***cuff tear arthropathy (CTA)****, and* ***CTA*** *remains the most common indication for RSA.* ***CTA*** *is a chronic condition, and most patients ultimately require operative treatment to improve function and provide pain relief; however, an initial trial of* ***nonoperative***

Sidebar 5-3

Transition words:

- First, second, third …
- Additionally
- However
- Thus
- Therefore
- Because
- Although
- Furthermore

treatment is typically warranted, including activity modification, anti-inflammatory medications, oral analgesics, corticosteroid injections, and gentle range of motion exercises. **Opioid** *medications are being used more commonly as a* **nonoperative** *modality to treat chronic musculoskeletal conditions, including osteoarthritis-associated pain. The use of* **opioid** *medications may lead to tolerance, hyperalgesia, and worse treatment outcomes.*[2]

The key is to find the critical words or phrases that are essential for the reader's understanding of the topic and then repeat them as necessary. But only use repetition as necessary, as too much repetition has been called *written clutter* and viewed as poor writing by the reader.

Exercise 4

Read the following passage and underline the key word(s) that are repeated for easier understanding.

Because active persons with an ACL injury who receive nonoperative care develop disabling knee conditions at a very high rate, reconstruction is often the recommended treatment. Some patients with an ACL injury want to delay their ACL reconstruction in order to complete a sports season or to make arrangements in their personal schedules (work, school, etc) to allow for surgery, rehabilitation, and recovery. Other patients may prefer to attempt nonoperative treatment before consenting to undergo ACL reconstruction. Certain other patients, referred to as "copers" by some authors, may be able to delay ACL reconstruction for months without having instability episodes or acquiring an additional knee injury. Such patients, however, are the exception; most patients will either have to modify their activities or receive surgical treatment to recover their functional ability.

Exercise 5

Read this famous quote often attributed to Abraham Lincoln. Does the repetitive word help or hinder understanding? Is it possible to rewrite the quote without repetition and without creating confusion?

"You can fool some of the people all of the time, and all of the people some of the time, but you cannot fool all of the people all of the time." —ascribed to Abraham Lincoln

Paragraph Readability and Text Justification

Some writers like the look of right-justified text with its crisp, even margins and think that it makes the manuscript more formal and thus more important. Many newspapers and books (even this one) use right justification. But many studies have shown that right-justified text is harder to read than left-justified text ("ragged" right edge) and a reader must read right-justified text at a significantly slower pace to equal comprehension of left-justified text.[4] This is caused by the brain having to work harder to read right-justified text due to the uneven spacing between words and hyphenation of words at the end of a line to make the margins equal. Additionally, the uniform look of right justification allows the eye to get lost more easily and slows down the reader even more. So the decision between left- and right-justified text comes down to the purpose of the writing. If the journal, publisher, or other authority requires one or the other, then authors must use their suggestion. But if the decision is up to the author, be nice to the reader and use left justification.

Changing Paragraph Structure and Content Through the Course of the Paper

When writing the manuscript, paragraph structure will change as the paper progresses. For example, the first paragraph of the introduction is usually quite broad in scope while the last paragraph of the introduction is specific to the study. Similarly, the first paragraph of the discussion is often used to summarize the results, while the last paragraph of the discussion may be a conclusions paragraph, which will summarize the whole study. Regardless, the mechanics of the paragraphs are still the same as each paragraph should be able to stand on its own, smoothly transition from paragraph to paragraph, and be consistent with terminology. In other words, despite a manuscript consisting of 20 or 30 individual paragraphs, each of which has a specific purpose in the paper, each paragraph still must follow the principles of strong paragraphs.

Turning Strong Paragraphs Into a Great Paper

Now that the techniques for writing strong paragraphs have been laid out, it is time to turn those paragraphs into a great paper. If following the outline from Chapter 2, the paragraphs should flow somewhat between topics and be logical in presentation. But something is always missing if one paragraph is simply stacked after another, and what is usually missing are transitions. Remember including transitions between sentences? The same techniques should be used to transition between paragraphs. Make sure each paragraph flows into the next one and that there is not a break in the logic or timeline between paragraphs.

After the paragraphs flow from one to the next, it is time to do some serious editing. This step is especially critical if different authors wrote different sections of the manuscript. The completed manuscript should be one cohesive document and the writing style should be consistent throughout. In my own writing, I often perform the statistics for the project, so I write the statistical analysis methods and the results section. Other authors on the paper will write the introduction, experiment methods, and the Discussion section. After everyone has submitted their sections, it is up to the lead author to assemble the paper in one writing style to be consistent throughout the paper. Failure to do this step well almost ensures a rejection letter from the journal. Every section is usually changed in some way to make a better overall paper. Do not take it personally if the lead author changes a particular author's work to improve clarity between sections. The lead author has a tough job editing, so be a good sport about the changes unless the message is drastically changed.

Conclusion

A strong paragraph is one unit of writing and can stand on its own. At a minimum, this requires a single topic and good paragraph structure—introductory sentence, supporting sentence(s), and then a concluding sentence. Other components such as the length, logical order, consistent terminology, transitions, and varying sentence structure all contribute to help create a strong paragraph. One, all, or none of the components can be used in strong paragraphs of a manuscript. After building strong paragraphs, an author will want to create the manuscript by linking the paragraphs together into sections and then linking the sections into the full manuscript. Remember that transitions make a paper flow from topic to topic so use them often. By incorporating some of the techniques in this chapter along with editing, an author can take strong paragraphs and turn them into a powerful manuscript.

References

1. O'Connor DP, Laughlin MS, Woods GW. Factors related to additional knee injuries after anterior cruciate ligament injury. *Arthroscopy*. 2005;21(4):431-438. doi:10.1016/j.arthro.2004.12.004.
2. Morris BJ, Laughlin MS, Elkousy HA, Gartsman GM, Edwards TB. Preoperative opioid use and outcomes after reverse shoulder arthroplasty. *J Shoulder Elb Surg*. 2015;24(1):11-16. doi:10.1016/j.jse.2014.05.002.
3. Morris BJ, Haigler RE, Cochran JM, et al. Obesity has minimal impact on short-term functional scores after reverse shoulder arthroplasty for rotator cuff tear arthropathy. *Am J Orthop (Belle Mead NJ)*. 2016;45(4):E180-E186.
4. Trollip SR, Sales G. Readability of computer-generated fill-justified text. *Human Factors*. 1986;28(2):159-163. doi:10.1177/001872088602800204.

Bibliography

Euchner C. *Sentences and Paragraphs: Mastering the Two Most Important Units of Writing*. Amazon Digital Services LLC; 2012.

Folse KS, Muchmore-Vokoun A, Solomon EV. *Great Paragraphs*. 3rd ed. Boston, MA: Heinle Cengage Learning; 2010.

Hofmann AH. *Scientific Writing and Communication: Papers, Proposals and Presentations*. New York, NY: Oxford University Press; 2010.

Kirszner LG, Mandell SR. *Focus on Writing*. 3rd ed. Boston, MA: Bedford/St. Martin's; 2014.

Strunk W Jr, White EB. *The Elements of Style*. 4th ed. Essex, England: Pearson Education Limited; 1999.

Zeiger M. *Essentials of Writing Biomedical Research Papers*. 2nd ed. New York, NY: McGraw Hill; 2000.

Chapter 6

Selecting a Journal and Navigating the *Author's Guide*

Mark Knoblauch, PhD, LAT, ATC, CSCS

Up until now, this book has focused on the foundations of writing, which includes issues such as designing a quality outline, sentence structure, and paragraph design. These concepts are key to effective writing, and a competent writer should have a have a strong understanding of each area when undertaking the process of manuscript development. When writing the manuscript, or in some cases even before writing the manuscript, it is essential that all authors have agreed on which journal they will pursue in order to publish their findings. Once a journal has been decided on, the manuscript should be formatted according to the submission requirements of the selected journal. For all journals, the submission guidelines found in the journal's *Author's Guide* outline the manuscript formatting and content requirements that must be met in order for that manuscript to be considered for publication. To get a manuscript sent out for review, each manuscript's authors must ensure that the submitted manuscript adheres to those guidelines outlined by the journal. Otherwise, the manuscript will likely be rejected outright before even critiquing the manuscript's content. This chapter provides insight into selecting an appropriate journal as well as an overview of the *Author's Guide*.

Selecting a Journal

Research stems from questions that a researcher investigates regarding a particular topic. If the involved researchers just wanted to know the answer for themselves, the results of their research could simply be locked up in a file cabinet, safe and sound from the critique of others. Such a situation is almost never the case, though. Rather, researchers strive to disseminate the results of their research to others in the field, which will in turn improve humankind's understanding of a particular topic and contribute to the overall body of knowledge that exists.

Conducting research and publishing the subsequent results are standard practice for most academics. Several options exist that allow a researcher to distribute their research findings

Knoblauch M. *Professional Writing in Kinesiology and Sports Medicine* (pp 53-67).
© 2019 Taylor & Francis Group.

including abstracts, reviews, monographs, peer-reviewed manuscripts, and book chapters. Factors that can influence which publishing options researchers might take include the stage at which one's research is at, time required for the research to get published, or even funding available. For example, preliminary findings of a major study may not be polished enough for a manuscript but may be suitable for a poster or abstract outlining the initial study findings. The choice for which avenue to pursue is often left to the researcher; however, promotion or even future hiring decisions can be most dependent upon a researcher showing evidence of peer-reviewed articles.[1] Therefore, pursuing journal publication may be the most relevant option for many researchers.

All medical journals have specific requirements regarding manuscript submissions. It is essential that authors understand these requirements prior to making a final journal selection. For example, if a journal has a word limit for a submission and a researcher's article is 30% longer than the word limit, it may be difficult to adequately revise the manuscript down to the word limit without losing vital portions of the manuscript's content. In such a case, the authors would be well-served to pursue publication in a different journal, particularly one with a higher word limit. Surprisingly, little research exists specific to journal selection. Knight and Steinbach[1] have outlined an approach that can work across disciplines and includes 5 major considerations that researchers should consider when deciding where to publish their research:

1. Likelihood of acceptance
2. Journal reputation
3. Journal visibility and potential article impact
4. Likelihood of timely publication
5. Philosophical and ethical issues

These 5 considerations should not be viewed as the only factors involved in journal selection, but they can provide insight to make the journal selection process more streamlined for manuscript authors.

Likelihood of Manuscript Acceptance

An important principle in deciding where a researcher should publish his or her research relates to the relevance between the research itself and the journal's scope. Most any journal website will outline that particular journal's scope or description, which describes the general research focus of publications released by that journal. For example, the journal *Sports Medicine* outlines their scope as the following:

> *Sports Medicine* focuses on definitive and comprehensive review articles that interpret and evaluate the current literature to provide the rationale for and application of research findings in the sports medicine and exercise field.

This description specifically summarizes the type of research that *Sports Medicine* publishes, and as such serves to outline the type of research manuscript that the journal seeks for publication. A researcher who feels that he or she has an outstanding case study would likely be unsuccessful in seeking to publish the case study in *Sports Medicine,* not because the case is poorly written but because *Sports Medicine* focuses on comprehensive review articles. In other words, the case study would simply be a poor fit for this one particular journal. Poor congruency between a submitted article's content and the journal's scope result in up to 10% of submissions being rejected prior to ever being sent out for review.[2]

Another way to assess an article's likelihood of acceptance is to evaluate the type of journals cited in the reference list of the researcher's pending submission.[1] Given that a manuscript is comprised of citations focused on a similar topic, a researcher may note a strong similarity of journals in his or her reference list. Or, he or she may note one particular journal's articles being cited repeatedly. This by no means indicates that a manuscript will be accepted to a particular journal, but this technique of reducing all possible journals down to those journals with a similar research focus can help save time as well as increase the likelihood of acceptance.

It is important to consider a manuscript's likelihood of acceptance, as there could be a significant financial impact even if a manuscript is ultimately rejected. Submission fees, though generally nominal ($50 to $100), may be required during the initial electronic submission process. Furthermore, color images published in an accepted manuscript can cost up to $1000 each. As will be discussed later, many journals have begun to offer manuscript authors an additional, though optional, fee that can exceed $3000 and serves to allow the accepted article to be offered as open access and available to any internet user. While publishing fees can begin to add up, all fees associated with publishing a manuscript in a particular journal will be outlined in the journal's *Author's Guide*. Therefore, authors should give strong consideration to a manuscript's likelihood of acceptance prior to submitting to a particular journal.

Journal Reputation

Publishing in a prestigious journal is a goal for all researchers. The inherent issues lies in determining just what makes a journal "prestigious." With little hesitation, most researchers will point to a journal's impact factor as an indicator of a journal's reputation. Traditionally, impact factor has been considered the standard for measuring a journal's prestige; however, in recent years, the use of impact factor for journal ranking has come under increased scrutiny specific to relevance and meaning of the impact factor.

Impact Factor

In its simplest terms, the impact factor is a numerical value assigned to a journal that is calculated from 2 values: the number of citations in the current year and the previous 2 years divided by the number of articles and reviews published in the same 2 years.[3] The impact factor was originally developed as an assessment tool so that publishers and librarians could manage inventory.[3,4] Over the years though, the impact factor has developed into a tool used by everyone from burgeoning researchers to tenure review committees as a way to assign a rank regarding the quality of a journal or quantifying its importance in science,[5] a transformation that even the originator of the impact factor, Eugene Garfield, himself regretted.[6]

Although the impact factor holds a reputation as the predominant journal ranking metric, it should be noted that the impact factor is by no means infallible. Garfield points out that rapidly changing fields could be weighted more if only including a single year of citations in the impact factor calculation. Conversely, more than 2 years of citations could be used, but this would in turn make an impact factor less current.[3]

Despite the perceived weaknesses in using impact factor as a gauge of a journal's reputation or prestige, the quality of a published article still today is dependent largely by the impact factor of the journal in which it is published.[5] In fact, the most often-asked question of any academic journal is "What's your impact factor?"[7] This may simply be due to the fact that there are no other widely accepted rubrics to judge the importance of a publication.[5]

Recently, the focus on impact factor has even progressed so far as to coin the phrase *impact factor mania*,[5,8] which represents the wasting of valuable time on the part of the researcher as well as reviewers brought about from overloading high-impact factor journals with submissions from researchers who are desperate to achieve a publication that would be viewed favorably during a professional review.[8] Interestingly, journals with high impact factors are often perceived from an opposing view—as having a low acceptance rate. This view creates a culture of exclusivity around that journal, in turn generating an assumption that articles published in that particular journal are of outstanding quality, which is not always justified.[5,9] General disdain surrounding impact factor among many scientists has led to efforts to effectively delegitimize its use including efforts to oppose using impact factors to assess individual researchers' work[7] as well as boycotting high-impact factor journals.[10]

Table 6-1. Impact Factors of Various Journals in the Fields of Kinesiology and Sports Medicine

JOURNAL	IMPACT FACTOR
Clinical Biomechanics	1.863
Exercise and Sport Sciences Reviews	5.065
Exercise Immunology Review	9.929
Gait & Posture	2.273
Human Movement Science	1.840
International Journal of Sports Medicine	2.453
Journal of Applied Physiology	3.257
Journal of Orthopaedic & Sports Physical Therapy	3.090
Journal of Sports Science and Medicine	1.990
The Journal of Strength and Conditioning Research	2.325
Medicine & Science in Sports & Exercise	4.141
Muscle & Nerve	2.496
Obesity	4.042
Physical Therapy	2.587
The Physician and Sportsmedicine	1.545
Research Quarterly for Exercise and Sport	2.268

Despite the appearance of overall criticism for the impact factor, it has been touted for its transparent aspect, cheap implementation, and value as an instantaneous measure of merit.[11] Though these reported benefits are arguable at best in light of the criticisms against the impact factor, it ultimately remains up to the researcher as to how much consideration impact factor should be given specific to the decision to publish in a particular journal. A list of impact factors (current at press time) for several sports medicine and kinesiology journals can be found in Table 6-1.

Journal Visibility

The rise of the internet has without a doubt changed the way that information can be accessed and disseminated. Both the quantity of information—through the rise of internet-based journals—as well as the simple access route to articles have contributed to the information warehouse that the internet has developed. The internet has provided an avenue that allows for publishing a manuscript online, which can provide a cheaper alternative to publishing in a printed journal. Yet, academics can be bombarded almost daily with emails soliciting anything from an invite to join the editorial board to near pleading for a submission of an article to a particular journal. While the increase in access to research information seems to have clear benefits, it is not without criticism.

Open-Access Publishing

Open-access journals have been described as those that participate in any publication arrangement in which content is available to readers online, in digital form, generally without charge or copyright restriction.[12] One reported benefit of open-access publishing is that it increases the exposure of a publication by simply being more easily available than a traditional article. This can be quantified indirectly by looking at the citations of open-access articles. One study looking at

> **Sidebar 6-1**
>
> Just how desperate can some of these "predatory" journals be? The television show *Adam Ruins Everything* once formatted an episode's script into a manuscript entitled "The Possible Irritating Effects of Nutritional Facts" and submitted it to the journal *Advances in Nutrition and Food Technology*. Upon receiving the required $369 publishing fee, the journal published the script of the show as though it were a scientific article—references and all! The article can be found at http://aeijst.in/The%20Possible%20Irritating%20Effects%20 of%20Nutritional%20Facts.pdf.

how open access affects citations found that among the disciplines of sociology, ecology, economics, and applied mathematics, 2280 (49%) open-access articles out of 4633 traditionally published articles had an average citation count of 9.04. Conversely, the remaining traditionally published journal articles had an average citation count of just 5.76.[13] Another study used article downloads and citations to evaluate the effect of free access. After evaluating more than 1600 articles in the field of psychology, the study found that full-text and PDF downloads along with unique visitors were 89%, 42%, and 23% higher, respectively, for open-access articles compared to subscription in the first 6 months after publication. However, citations were no higher for open access than for subscription-based articles.[14]

The evidence of higher downloads but no noticeable increase in citations is noteworthy for a researcher considering open-access publishing. The higher downloads reported for open-access articles suggests higher visibility for the articles published online. However, the fact that open-access articles are not cited at a higher rate than subscription-based journals could be an indicator of the perceived quality of open-access articles. For many scholars, the benefit of open-access journals appears mixed. Positive aspects of open-access articles reported by academics include improved and more equitable access to knowledge as well as increased availability of research papers to the developing world. Furthermore, open access provides faster publication times as well as reduction in financial costs associated with journal subscriptions and time savings specific to photocopying and interlibrary loans.[15]

However, not all academics favor the open-access approach. Jeffrey Beall, an academic librarian, noticed the extensive amount of spam mail he was receiving from sites inviting him to submit a journal article. Upon investigation, he noted that " … many of these publishers have a low article acceptance threshold, with a false-front or non-existent peer review process. Unlike professional publishing operations, whether subscription-based or ethically sound open access, these predatory publishers add little value to scholarship, pay little attention to digital preservation, and operate using fly-by-night, unsustainable business models."[16] Beall even goes so far as to publish a list of open-access journals that identifies "predator" journals,[17] which he classified as "those that unprofessionally exploit the author-pays model of open-access publishing (ie, "gold open access") for their own profit. Typically, these publishers spam professional email lists, broadly soliciting article submissions for the clear purpose of gaining additional income." This is not to say that all open-access publishers are predatory. In fact, an online database entitled the *Directory of Open-Access Journals,* contrary to Beall's "predatory" list, identifies "high-quality" open-access journals and can be found at https://doaj.org (Sidebar 6-1).

The decision of whether to publish an article using the traditional printed journal approach or via open access is ultimately the choice of the researcher. As shown previously, the debate regarding open-access publication has not been settled. Specific to journal visibility though, open access vs traditional publishing should not be the only factor involved. Journal visibility has been described as "including subscription base and whether the regular readership is homogenous and includes the people you want to impact."[18] Written differently, journal visibility could be argued to be more about whether the readership of the journal matches the intent of the submitted manuscript, because those who have an interest in the manuscript's topic are obviously more likely to read the manuscript. For example, a researcher who reveals that curcumin has an effect on athletic endurance may be better served by submitting the manuscript to *The Journal of Strength and Conditioning Research* than the *Journal of Herbs, Spices, and Medicinal Plants* because in this case, the outcome—a positive effect on endurance—would likely generate a more focused readership in a conditioning journal than the variable—curcumin—might generate in a herbalism journal. Therefore, it could be expected that the manuscript's visibility would be higher—and the target audience more relevant—in a conditioning journal.

Likelihood of Timely Publication

Whereas the goal of any submitted manuscript is to achieve publication, the timeline by which that publication occurs could be an important factor. As discussed previously, the relatively rapid nature by which open-access publications are available to the public can be a factor that sways some researchers to pursue open-access publication, even with the peer-review process required for many open-access journals. If choosing the traditional printed journal route, however, the timeframe for publication should be considered as the time until the accepted article has been assigned to an issue and is either available online or is printed in the issue. Many traditional journal's articles are available online for a fee prior to publication in the printed journal. The online version of the article will be assigned a designation of "published online date" weeks or months before being assigned to a specific journal issue that includes page numbers.

Throughout the process to publication, several events factor into how long before an article is accessible including the time required for peer review of the article, the number of review cycles and subsequent revisions, the review of page proofs, and copy editing. Furthermore, a backlog of accepted articles awaiting publication in a printed journal can be a year or more.[1] When coupled with the journal's publication rate, or how often a journal publishes an issue per year, an accepted, proofed article can likely have a significant "wait" time before being fully published.

Understanding the time frame required for an article's full publication is important for authors considering publication in a traditional journal. For example, submitting to a journal with a longer response rate may influence a tenure and promotion portfolio, especially if a deadline is approaching. Separately, when 2 researchers are independently working on the same significant research problem, the first author to get a subsequent article published will likely receive the majority of accolades. If an important deadline must be reached regarding a manuscript's publication, open-access publishing may be a viable option for the researcher (Sidebar 6-2).

Philosophical and Ethical Issues

Knight and Steinbach focus this value regarding journal selection largely on choosing open-access or traditional journal publication, as detailed at length earlier. However, the researcher may take issue with other philosophical issues, such as the peer-review process and to what level it occurs with a particular journal.

Peer Review

Peer review has been defined as the evaluation of research findings for competence, significance, and originality by qualified experts[19] and consists of a structured process that functions to ensure the quality of scientific information.[20] This expert (ie, "peer") review is designed to ensure that the research conducted in the manuscript is of a quality that ensures that the findings reported are meaningful. While peer review is almost universally accepted as a process that improves and ensures research quality, it is not without its shortcomings. Limitations of peer review include a potential for bias toward certain researchers, an inability to expose research flaws, unexpected delays in publication, and no clear system that ensures that peer review detects

Sidebar 6-2

Does getting something published first really matter, as long as the facts show that something has been discovered? Most will probably argue that publication does indeed matter, since a discovery sitting on someone's desk does little to aid humankind until the information is disseminated.

Perhaps the most poignant story illustrating this effect can be told in the controversy between Isaac Newton and Gottfried Wilhelm von Leibniz over the discovery of calculus. Newton's discovery of calculus was documented as having occurred first, during the years of 1664 to 1666. Leibniz, on the other hand, reportedly discovered his somewhat less complicated version of calculus between 1672 and 1676. Newton made the choice to table his discovery, not publishing his findings until 1693. Leibniz, however, published his findings in 1684 and 1686, nearly a decade before Newton. A battle ensued, with public outcry accusing Leibniz of stealing Newton's findings and claiming them for his own. Eventually the matter was taken to court in 1711, and the Royal Society—of which Newton was the president—eventually found Leibniz guilty of plagiarism. It was only years later, after Leibniz's death, that it was eventually realized that the 2 scientists had discovered calculus independently.

Though a classic story, the controversy between Newton and Leibniz illustrates what researchers still encounter today. Whereas research should not duplicate something that has already been discovered, what defines "discovery"? Furthermore, at what stage in the research process does a new finding become official? Lab tests provide data, but that data must be analyzed. That analysis must then be described in the context of how it applies to the real world. And finally, the application of the data along with all components of the scientific process used to rationalize the experiment must hold up to peer review. Even then, a peer-accepted article may be delayed months or potentially years before finally being published. Only then do the results of an experiment become public knowledge, or perhaps in the minds of some, become discovered. Using that mindset, it could be argued that among 2 researchers investigating the same phenomenon, the researcher who gets his or her work to print first will be credited with the discovery. The other will forever be thought of having researched something that is already known. So, does time to publication matter—most would respond with an emphatic **yes**!

scientific misconduct.[2] Despite its imperfections, the process of peer review plays an essential role in manuscript publication.[2]

The process of peer review involves the author, the journal editor, and multiple manuscript reviewers and can take one of several routes. Open review is a process where both the author and reviewer identities are known to each other. Single-blind reviews involve the process by which the reviewer's identity is hidden, and is the most common form of review.[21] Double-blind reviews are such that both the author and reviewer identities are unknown to each other. At least one study reports that double-blind reviews are the preferred review method by academics.[22]

Although designed as a tool to ensure that new research is of a high quality, peer review does have shortcomings in the way of potential bias. Bias represents unfair favoritism for or against a particular thing, and in research that "thing" could range from a particular research topic to a particular researcher. In peer review, reviewers may feel that a particular author's name is established enough to favor acceptance of a submitted manuscript. Or, a manuscript may be rejected simply because there was only one author, or the manuscript came from a relatively small institution, or because the manuscript did not find significant results. Table 6-2 outlines various types of bias associated with the peer-review process.[21]

Table 6-2. Real or Perceived Forms of Bias in Peer Review

BIAS AS A FUNCTION OF AUTHOR CHARACTERISTICS

Affiliation bias	Researchers and reviewers have formal or informal working relationships
Nationality bias	Nationality of the researcher can influence a manuscript's or grant application's acceptance
Prestige bias	Researchers with higher prestige disproportionally obtain resources such as grants, awards, etc, that in turn predispose the researcher to additional prestige
Language bias	Primary language of the author's country can affect manuscript acceptance
Gender bias	Men and women are treated differently in peer review

BIAS AS A FUNCTION OF REVIEWER CHARACTERISTICS

Content-based bias	Partiality for or against a manuscript based on its methods, theory, results, etc
Confirmation bias	Favorably viewing results that support a view while unfavorably viewing results that do not support a particular view
Conservatism bias	A propensity to unfavorably view new or groundbreaking research
Interdisciplinary bias	Unfavorably viewing a manuscript that spans more than one specific area of research
Publication bias	A tendency to publish research that demonstrates favorable (eg, significant) outcomes rather than negative

Electronic Options for Finding a Journal

As discussed, finding the best journal to which an author should submit a manuscript requires several considerations. Over the past few years, electronic tools have been developed to assist researchers in selecting the best journal for their manuscript. These tools require rather basic information such as a subject area and abstract, and can even allow the researcher to choose whether to limit results to open-access journals. For example, the Journal/Author Name Estimator (JANE) is an online tool that suggests relevant journals to which a researcher may wish to submit a manuscript. Search results on some of these websites can then be stratified by the manuscript author based on impact factor or expected review time.

Navigating the Journal's Manuscript Submission Guidelines

Publication of any manuscript requires submission to and ultimately acceptance by a journal. In 2014, there were more than 2.5 million articles in science, technology, and medicine published in more than 28,000 journals.[23] The high number of journals indicates that manuscript authors have a wealth of relevant journals to which to submit their work. The selection of the appropriate journal, however, is not a stand-alone aspect in the path to publication. Rather, it is a component that must be incorporated into the drafting of the manuscript itself.

To get published, an author must draft a manuscript with information essential for others to understand the rationale, methods, results, and implications of the research conducted. Without

Table 6-3. Manuscript Formatting Requirements Across Several Sports Medicine and Kinesiology Journals

JOURNAL	TITLE LENGTH	ABSTRACT LENGTH	KEY WORDS LIMIT	MAXIMUM TEXT (ORIGINAL ARTICLE)	MAXIMUM REFERENCES
The American Journal of Sports Medicine	N/A	350	4	6000	60
Gait & Posture	N/A	300	6	3000	30
Journal of Athletic Training	16 words	300	3	N/A	30
Journal of Rehabilitation Medicine	N/A	200	5	2500	40
Journal of Science and Medicine in Sport	N/A	350	6	3000	30
Journal of Sport and Health Science	20 words	250	8	5000	N/A
Muscle & Nerve	80 spaces	150	5	4000	No limit
Physical Therapy	150 characters	275	N/A	4000	75
The Physician and Sportsmedicine	120 characters	300	10	6000	30 minimum

these components the manuscript is effectively meaningless as the complete message intended by the research cannot be conveyed. However, the drafting of the original manuscript must also take into account the style and formatting requirements of the journal to which the manuscript will be submitted, and it is essential that manuscript authors be aware of these requirements early in the manuscript writing process.

Essentially all journals include a set of guidelines that submitted manuscripts must adhere to in the form of an *Author's Guide, Submission Guidelines, Instructions for Authors*, or similarly named section. These guidelines outline the format, style, and order of the manuscript and must be adhered to in order for a submission to get to the review phase. Therefore, failing to identify a target journal early in the research process can result in time-consuming revisions and formatting updates to get the manuscript into the layout required by a particular journal. For example, formats differ among journals specific to abstract word limits, title length, font required, section headings, and table/image requirements. Table 6-3 outlines the formatting requirements listed by several journals in the field of sports medicine and kinesiology. It is key to format a prepared manuscript according to these requirements as an improperly formatted manuscript can result in outright rejection by the target journal.

Accessing a journal's submission guidelines is relatively easy in this digital age. Researchers need only to navigate to the journal's homepage, find the link entitled "Information for Authors" (or similar), and click. Authors will then be directed to a webpage that outlines the procedures and styles required of a manuscript prior to final submission to the journal. The content of the submission guidelines differs for each journal and can range from rather general to highly detailed. An outline of the general sections one can expect to find in the submission guidelines is discussed in the following pages.

Author Guidelines Components

Submitting an article for publication allows a journal the rights to publish an author's work. In turn, most journals request certain assurances from the manuscript author. These assurances focus on several legal and ethical perspectives such as addressing potential conflicts of interest, adherence to ethical standards, or copyright assignment. Furthermore, it should be expected that a submitted manuscript will not advance through the review process without all necessary forms on file with the journal of interest, as these forms are the author's declaration that the submitted manuscript adheres to the journal's basic requirements. Several examples of expected forms or assurances that are required with a manuscript submission follow. This is not meant to be an exhaustive list, but rather outlines the most common required forms.

Conflict of Interest Form

Many researchers have established focused research tracks that establish their expertise in a particular area. For most, their research findings improve upon what is already known and improve the greater good with no direct benefit back to the researcher. However, it is possible that a researcher is conducting research that, if favorable results are found, could benefit him or her directly in a variety of ways, one of which could include financial gain. While is it well-known that much of the research conducted will eventually lead to financial gain at some point (eg, drug or product sales), an issue arises when a researcher is financially linked to a particular research outcome. This in effect creates a conflict between the researcher and the outcome and in turn invites a viable opportunity for bias. Conflict of interest forms openly reveal these potential relationships and allow the journal editor or—if the conflict does not prevent publication—the reader to make his or her own decision as to whether the article and its outcomes are valid in light of the reported conflict.

Journals will require either inserting text into a manuscript that outlines the presence or lack of a conflict, or completion of a separate conflict of interest form that must be submitted with the manuscript. Researchers bear the responsibility of reporting whether a relationship they hold with a particular entity could be considered a conflict. Generally, conflicts center on the research outcome itself. Therefore, receiving free supplies or equipment used for conducting the research would not likely be considered a conflict as long as the outcomes of the research are not influenced by the gifting of those items. In fact, this very process happens quite often, as companies will contact a researcher and agree to provide their new product along with a set amount of funding to allow the researcher to test the effectiveness of their product. This does not constitute any conflict assuming that the researcher is independent (eg, not employed, a stockholder, etc) of the company and does not gain financially from the research outcomes he or she reports.

Conflicts of interest are largely based on perception, and in the case of manuscripts, this perception will often be determined by the reader. One technique to help determine whether a particular relationship could be construed as a conflict is for the researcher to ask whether an exposed relationship of some kind between the researcher and the company might alter the reader's view of the research outcomes. If so, the researcher would be recommended to report the potential conflict. This does not change the outcome of the research but rather provides relevant information to the reader that in turn allows the reader to determine whether the conflict may influence his or her interpretation of the outcomes.

Sample Problem A

A company, "HyperGrowth," contacts a researcher who has an established line of research investigating the effects of skeletal muscle response to electrical stimulation. The company claims to have designed a product consumers can wear under their clothing that will provide continued electrical stimulation sufficient to induce muscle hypertrophy over a relatively short period of time. HyperGrowth offers the researcher $20,000 in funding and 5 muscle stimulation units to conduct a research study investigating their claims.

In their introductory email, HyperGrowth requests that they as a company be allowed to serve as a content editor of any manuscripts prior to the manuscript being sent out for peer review. If the researcher adheres to HyperGrowth's request, do you feel this represents a conflict of interest for any manuscripts that result from testing the effects of this muscle stimulator?

Sample Problem B

A researcher has a history of experiencing heat exhaustion during endurance running events in which she participated. She found literature about a specific herbal product that showed benefits in maintaining a lower core body temperature in military members of a foreign nation. She conducted sound research that showed a benefit in reducing core temperature in trained endurance athletes, and would like to test the effects of the herbal product in reducing heat exhaustion incidence in endurance athletes. Given her own status as an endurance competitor, do you feel her research findings showing a benefit of the herbal product on reducing the incidence of heat exhaustion to be a conflict of interest?

Ethical Adherence

In 1997, a group of journal editors formed the Committee on Publication Ethics (COPE), which serves to provide advice on publication ethics as well as assist in handling research and publication misconduct. The committee developed a document entitled *Code of Conduct and Best Practice Guidelines for Journal Editors*, which provides a set of standards to which individual COPE members are expected to adhere. These guidelines are the culmination of requests from journal editors specific to various aspects of publishing, such as journal editors' general duties, relationship with reviewers, and dealing with misconduct, and provide best practice recommendations for how to address these and other various issues. Many journals now require that with a manuscript submission, the submitting author must acknowledge agreement with a particular journal's position on publication ethics, usually outlined by the COPE document.

Copyright Assignment

The rights to any manuscript can be held by any person or institution. Should a manuscript be developed yet remain unpublished, that copyright is held for the life of the author plus an additional 70, 95, or 120 years, depending on the makeup of authorship.[24] Since most authors develop manuscripts with the intention of achieving publication, the copyright laws relating to unpublished work is irrelevant. With submission of a manuscript, it is important for authors to understand that the rights to that manuscript are at issue. Therefore, journals have outlined their policy specific to the manuscript's copyright in some form of a *Copyright Assignment* document (Sidebar 6-3).

Numerous journals allow authors to retain copyright upon article submission. These authors are, in effect, granting a license to the journal to publish that manuscript while still retaining the rights to the manuscript. By retaining the rights to their own article, manuscript authors can in most cases continue to use the article without first contacting the publishing journal. Conversely, retaining a manuscript's rights does not occur when the authors assign copyright to the journal as is required for many journals. At that point, usually upon publication of the article, the journal owns rights to the article and the authors must obtain permission to use the article, outside of certain provisions set out by the journal such as internal use in an author's classroom.

Author Contributions

Achieving publication of an article is a major accomplishment for all manuscript authors and can have a positive impact for each author specific to promotion/tenure, salary, job status, etc. Therefore, simply being listed as an author may provide a significant benefit for a researcher. This has in turn invited problems of its own. "Coercive authorship" and the "White Bull effect" are authorship abuse concepts that have been used to outline the assignment of authorship for individuals in response to their exertion of seniority or supervisory status over subordinates and

Sidebar 6-3

Although copyright law is designed to protect authors of unpublished work, what happens when one member of several authors decides to pursue publication without express agreement from all other authors? This was the premise of a 2015 legal case, Mallon vs Marshall. In 2008, Andrew Mallon went to work in John Marshall's lab as a postdoctoral associate at Brown University. The pair, along with 5 other authors, eventually submitted a manuscript to *Neuron* that outlined their work with a drug designed to affect memory disorders.

Neuron ultimately rejected the submission in late 2011, and the 2 discussed other journals to consider for resubmission, including *PLoS Biology*. However, the collaboration between Mallon and Marshall had fallen apart around that same time. Mallon eventually left Brown University, and there was no contact between Mallon and Marshall for over 15 months. During that time, Marshall had contacted a new collaborator, Dennis Goebel, and throughout 2012 the original manuscript was revised and resubmitted through several rejections. Eventually, a heavily revised version was accepted in 2013 which did not include Mallon as an author but instead noted him in the acknowledgments.

Mallon eventually filed a lawsuit to receive co-authorship and copyright of the accepted article, and a full retraction of the accepted article. The basis for Mallon's argument was case law stating that "the authors of a joint work are co-owners of copyright in the work," and Mallon felt that as a co-author of the original manuscript he maintains copyright to the published article. However, the Copyright Act holds that "where a work is prepared over a period of time, the portion of it that has been fixed at any particular time constitutes the work as of that time, and where the work has been prepared in different versions, each version constitutes a separate work." Marshall and Goebel's claim was that since Mallon left the lab, there was no longer an intent to create a joint work with him and the revised and ultimately published manuscript was in effect a new submission. Eventually, this argument was accepted and the court ended up siding with Marshall.

junior investigators without appropriate contribution.[25] However, coercion is not the only form of authorship abuse. Honorary authorship results from granting authorship out of respect, or in an attempt to add legitimacy to a manuscript without the requisite manuscript contribution from the recipient. The ethics of determining the order and contributors to the author list are outlined in greater detail later in Chapter 14.

Traditionally, manuscript author lists did not outline the contributions each author made to a particular published article, and there was no effective way to ensure that each author listed made a significant contribution to a manuscript. In contrast, anyone who has watched movie credits roll at the end are aware of the precise role that each credited person performed for a particular film. It is not unusual to have a single author on a manuscript for a relatively concise experiment. What can be somewhat problematic is to establish the contributions of each author when the list expands to 10 or maybe 15 authors (or in certain fields, author lists of up to 5000[26]). To help provide a standard for reporting author contributions, the International Committee of Medical Journal Editors (ICMJE) recommends that 4 criteria be met for each contributing author (ICMJE.org):

- Substantial contributions to the conception or design of the work; or the acquisition, analysis, or interpretation of data for the work; AND
- Drafting the work or revising it critically for important intellectual content; AND
- Final approval of the version to be published; AND
- Agreement to be accountable for all aspects of the work in ensuring that questions related to the accuracy or integrity of any part of the work are appropriately investigated and resolved.

Many journals now require that all manuscript authors provide written acknowledgment of meeting these criteria before a submission is considered for review.

For individuals who do not meet each of the qualifications listed above, it is recommended that the individual be recognized via an acknowledgment rather than as an author. Therefore, an individual who helped log or analyze data but did not serve a role in drafting, revising, or giving final approval of the manuscript would be better suited for an acknowledgment than authorship. However, the ICMJE points out that acknowledging an individual for his or her contributions to a manuscript implies that individual's endorsement of the manuscript's outcomes. Because of this implied endorsement, it is recommended that all acknowledged individuals provide written permission to be acknowledged prior to submission of the manuscript.

Defining the Study's Design

Most journals require the submitting author to identify the study design that is associated with his or her article. It is imperative that the study design is established prior to writing the manuscript, as formatting requirements typically differ between study designs even within the same journal. Failing to identify the appropriate study design as well as the intended journal can result in a significant amount of manuscript editing required to meet the journal's submission guidelines. Common study designs include:

- Original research/randomized control trial: Collection of data using fieldwork, surveys, interviews, or observation that undergoes formal collection and analysis
- Meta-analysis: A summation of several studies that statistically tests the pooled data
- Systematic review: A summation of several studies on a centralized topic that includes inclusion and exclusion criteria for related studies
- Crossover design: All treatments are applied to all participants at various points throughout the study; in effect, participants "cross over" from one treatment to another throughout the experiment
- Cohort study: One group with a disease are matched with a group of nondiseased individuals and followed over time
- Case-control study: A study used to determine if an exposure is associated with an outcome such as disease by following 2 groups, 1 with a disease and 1 without a disease
- Cross-sectional study: Identifying particular characteristics of a population at a single point in time, or in some cases at particular intervals over time
- Case series: Following a group of diseased subjects over time and reporting their outcomes
- Case report: Identifying outcomes from a single individual or in some cases a single event (eg, football game) or location (eg, high school)
- Descriptive epidemiology study: Reporting events (eg, injuries) associated with a particular event
- Controlled laboratory study: An in vitro or in vivo study that statistically analyzes the results from an experimental and a control group
- Descriptive laboratory study: An in vitro or in vivo study that provides descriptive characteristics such as a new event, anatomy, or physiology

Once the study design is selected, the manuscript can be formatted according to the specific requirements outlined for that study design. It should be noted that for some journals, case reports may also require a separate signed release form from the patient prior to a manuscript being sent out for review.

Manuscript Style Elements

Before the submitted manuscript is sent out for peer review, it is checked for compliance with the journal's submission guidelines. Rejection of a submitted manuscript based on something as minor as an incorrect font or inappropriate margins is possible; therefore, it is essential that manuscript authors take the time to ensure that their work is compatible with the requirements of the particular journal to which they are submitting the manuscript. Just as there are a vast number of journals that publish articles in a particular field, there are also ample submission requirements for those journals. As such, the intricacies of all journal formatting requirements will not be discussed here. Instead, the reader is referred to Table 6-3 to show how each journal can have individual formatting requirements, and it is essential for manuscript authors to review these style (eg, font, font size, spacing, line numbering, etc) and wording (eg, title, abstract, and manuscript word count maximums) requirements carefully.

Tables and Images

One particular area that formatting requirements are essential is in the area of tables and image preparation. Tables are usually generated within a word processing document from analyzed data and are relatively easy to format. Images, however, can be more complicated in that the quality in which an original image is saved must be adequate for the journal requirements.

Dots per inch, or "DPI", is an antiquated but still-used measure of printer resolution. Journal requirements for image DPI differ, but halftone (ie, greyscale) image requirements are often in the 200 to 300 DPI range. It is vital that prior to labeling or manipulating an image, the original image is saved and only copies of that image are manipulated. Otherwise, if an author happened to save an original image at a lower resolution than required, the lower image quality would be rejected by the journal and thereby require a new image to be captured. By using only copies of the original image there is effectively endless leeway in manipulating the image.

Manuscript authors should also become adept at using image "layers," which can save valuable time when reformatting images for submission to a different journal. Creating image panels, or a collection of individual images positioned to create a single new image, can be time consuming. By creating and saving a panel in layers, one small change to the panel does not necessitate completely refabricating the entire panel; rather, the change can be made at a point in which only that layer was affected and all previous layers will remain unaffected. This can be particularly helpful when submitting a rejected manuscript to a different journal, as the panel's image alignment and content can be maintained while having to only change minor details such as the text that identifies each image in the panel.

Resubmissions

Because formatting guidelines are specific to each journal, in the unfortunate event that a manuscript is rejected by one journal, it likely cannot simply be resubmitted to another journal. Rather, the manuscript will need to undergo substantial reformatting to maintain compliance with the second journal's manuscript guidelines. Therefore, the formatting process starts anew for a manuscript each time it is resubmitted to a new journal. The reorganization likely applies to whole sections of the manuscript as it is possible that the second journal's requirements may include vastly different section headings than the original submission. For example, a journal that rejected the initial submission of a manuscript may have required a Discussion section, while a second journal mandates separate Discussion, Conclusion, and Clinical Implications sections. The authors would then have to extract material from the original manuscript's Discussion section and format that text into suitable text for the Conclusion and Implications sections. Such movement of text may or may not require additional manuscript writing as well, or could require removal of substantial amounts of text if the new journal's word limit is less than that of the original journal.

More information on adapting a manuscript's content for these specific sections is presented in Chapter 10.

References and Citations

It should also be expected that each journal will have specific reference and citation requirements for a potential manuscript. The author guidelines for each journal will outline the reference style required as well as the format required for citations within the manuscript (eg, numeric or author/date). Typically, the *Author's Guide* will refer the author to one of several guides such as the *AMA Manual of Style* for assistance with referencing and may or may not provide citation and reference examples. Therefore, the *Author's Guide* requirements for referencing and citing previous work will not be outlined here. However, manuscript authors should be aware that some citation programs such as Endnote include reference and citation templates for specific journals. This option can save significant time for the author when preparing a manuscript. More detailed information on referencing can be found in Chapter 8.

References

1. Knight L, Steinbach T. Selecting an appropriate publication outlet: a comprehensive model of journal selection criteria for researchers in a broad range of academic disciplines. *International Journal of Doctoral Studies*. 2008;3:59-78.
2. Benos DJ, Bashari E, Chaves JM, et al. The ups and downs of peer review. *Advances in Physiology Education*. 2007;31(2):145-152.
3. Garfield E. The history and meaning of the journal impact factor. *JAMA*. 2006;295(1):90-93.
4. Moustafa K. The disaster of the impact factor. *Science and Engineering Ethics*. 2015;21(1):139-142.
5. Casadevall A, Fang FC. Causes for the persistence of impact factor mania. *mxBio*. 2014;5(2):e00064-14.
6. Garfield E. Journal impact factor: a brief review. *CMAJ*. 1999;161(8):979-980.
7. Schekman R, Patterson M. Reforming research assessment. *Elife*. 2013;2:e00855.
8. Alberts B. Impact factor distortions. *Science*. 2013;340(6134):787.
9. Petsko GA. The one new journal we might actually need. *Genome Biology*. 2011;12(9):129.
10. Schekman R. How journals like Nature, Cell and Science are damaging science. *The Guardian*. 2013;9:12-23.
11. Eyre-Walker A, Stoletzki N. The assessment of science: the relative merits of post-publication review, the impact factor, and the number of citations. *PLoS Biol*. 2013;11(10):e1001675.
12. Salem DN, Boumil MM. Conflict of interest in open-access publishing. *N Engl J Med*. 2013;369(5):491.
13. Norris M, Oppenheim C, Rowland F. The citation advantage of open-access articles. *Journal of the American Society for Information Science and Technology*. 2008;59(12):1963-1972.
14. Davis PM, Lewenstein BV, Simon DH, Booth JG, Connolly MJL. Open access publishing, article downloads, and citations: randomised controlled trial. *BMJ*. 2008;337:a568.
15. Togia A, Korobili S. Attitudes towards open access: a meta-synthesis of the empirical literature. *Information Services & Use*. 2014;34(3-4):221-231.
16. Haug C. The downside of open-access publishing. *N Engl J Med*. 2013;368(9):791-793.
17. Beall J. *Beall's list of predatory publishers 2013*. Scholarly Open Access. 2012.
18. Thompson B. Publishing your research results: some suggestions and counsel. *Journal of Counseling and Development*. 1995;73(3):342.
19. Brown T. *Peer Review and the Acceptance of New Scientific Ideas*. London, England: Sense About Science; 2004.
20. Macrina FL, ed. *Scientific Integrity: Text and Cases in Responsible Conduct of Research*. Washington, DC: ASM Press; 2005:61-90.
21. Lee CJ, Sugimoto CR, Zhang G, Cronin B. Bias in peer review. *Journal of the American Society for Information Science and Technology*. 2013;64(1):2-17.
22. Ware M. Peer review in scholarly journals: perspective of the scholarly community—results from an international study. *Information Services & Use*. 2008;28(2):109-112.
23. Ware M, Mabe M. *The STM Report: An Overview of Scientific and Scholarly Journal Publishing*. The Hague, Netherlands: International Association of Scientific, Technical and Medical Publishers; 2015.
24. Office. U.S.C. Duration of Copyright. 2011.
25. Strange K. Authorship: why not just toss a coin? *American Journal of Physiology-Cell Physiology*. 2008;295(3): C567-C575.
26. Aad G, Abbott B, Abdallah J, et al. Combined Measurement of the Higgs Boson Mass in p p Collisions at s= 7 and 8 TeV with the ATLAS and CMS Experiments. *Physical Review Letters*. 2015;114(19):191803.

Chapter 7

Creating the "Hook"
Drafting an Effective Title and Abstract

Mark Knoblauch, PhD, LAT, ATC, CSCS and Josh Yellen, EdD, LAT, ATC

The Power of the Manuscript Title

For having so few words, a manuscript title exerts quite an influence. In a precious 10 to 15 words, a manuscript title must orient the reader to the manuscript's topic, highlight the purpose or findings of the associated research, and contain appropriate key words that can be recognized by search engines, all while serving to motivate the reader to delve deeper into the article. A poorly written title could easily be the downfall of an outstanding manuscript, as complicated search engine algorithms may inadvertently pass over an important article when a relevant search is conducted. Such failure of an article to show up in the search results reduces the article's impact on the medical community.[1] Similarly, a title written with too much detail could appear limited in its overall scope. Or, a title written with too many acronyms may simply come across as confusing. Thus, a clear and comprehensive title is an essential component of a well-crafted manuscript.

The Importance of an Effective Title

The phrase "You never get a second chance to make a first impression" could easily describe the mantra for an effective manuscript title. Think about this—prospective peer reviewers may be provided only the title when initially asked their interest in reviewing a paper, and the decision to review or decline the manuscript is therefore based solely on the clarity of the title.[1] Some consider an effective title to be a statement of the aim of the manuscript's work.[2] Whereas research aims outline the overall purpose of a study, it should be expected for the title to convey a similar message. A title that is confusing, cramped, or too generic will fail to provide the interest necessary to draw in the reader. In a perfect world, the title should stimulate enough interest to direct the reader to the abstract, which in turn motivates him or her toward reading the full article. Unfortunately, poor or confusing design of some manuscript titles can provide just enough information to confuse the reader, in turn forcing him or her to scan the abstract to determine whether the article is relevant.

Knoblauch M. *Professional Writing in Kinesiology and Sports Medicine* (pp 69-76).
© 2019 Taylor & Francis Group.

The title is the first component of a published article that a reader will see. As such, the title has a vital role in providing the first impression of the article and can in turn contribute to the manuscript's readership.[3] For most researchers, their first exposure to an article occurs when an internet search is conducted. Relevant search results are returned in the form of a list of 10 to 20 titles (along with snippets of the abstract) per search page. This is where the first impression of a title is most important, as titles from the most relevant articles must stand out from all other titles returned in the web results. The researcher will most likely engage in title scanning while looking for relevance to his or her intended topic.[4] Because titles are quickly scanned, those titles that are succinct, informative, and somewhat catchy while remaining pertinent to the researcher's topic will have a better chance of being accessed.

How **Not** to Write a Title

Before outlining the steps in drafting an effective title, it might be relevant to point out how not to write a manuscript title. Despite the importance of the title, there are no set requirements or standards for how to write a manuscript title other than what may be outlined specific to word or character counts in each journal's *Author's Guide* (see Chapter 6). The lack of formal rules for drafting a title could lead one to think that there is no such thing as a "wrong" title. While true, there are certainly "bad" or "ineffective" titles.

Titles Written as Questions

Manuscript titles written as a question are generally not recommended,[5] even though they do still occur in the literature. Some authors counter that organizing a title as a question might in fact motivate the reader to read the full text to establish the author's answer to the question,[6] while those opposed to question-based manuscript titles further suggest that doing so reduces the article's likelihood of being retrieved during an electronic query because the specific study topic is not explicitly outlined.[7] Consider the following title posed as a question:

Does pre-activity quadriceps stretching affect vertical jump power generation?

Posing the title as a question contradicts the entire purpose of the study, which is to in fact answer the very question posed by the title. If the author takes away the question word (ie, "does"), the remaining phrase almost becomes a title itself, needing only a directional lead such as changing "affect" to "affects" in order to convey not only the purpose but also the results of the study.

Extraneous Words in Titles

As discussed, titles often have a word or character limit that is established by the respective journal. Adding extraneous words not inherent to the research itself can cause a title to exceed the established word limit, not to mention distract the reader from the intent of the research article. Consider the following title:

An investigation into the influence of therapeutic ultrasound on pre-activity muscle warming

The words "an investigation into" are irrelevant to the title and only serve to contribute additional words and characters without strengthening the intended message of the title. Whereas the manuscript itself is outlining a scientific study, it is already established that a scientific study or investigation has been conducted; therefore, any mention of that would simply be repetitive and unnecessary. By removing those unnecessary words, the title becomes "the influence of therapeutic ultrasound on pre-activity muscle warming," which sounds very much like a well-designed study aim that effectively doubles as an effective manuscript title. By removing the extraneous words, more detail could then be added to further strengthen the title (eg, "in elite high jumpers").

Along the same lines as using excessive words, it is generally recommended to avoid composing titles as complete sentences. Titles should be grammatically correct no matter their length, but a degree of poetic license exists in manuscript title drafting that forgives authors who generate effective titles that end up as sentence fragments. This allowance of fragmented titles is in large part due to the various word or character limits set out by a particular journal. For instance, an eloquently written, grammatically correct manuscript title could be written as:

Athletes who suffer lateral ankle sprains are more likely to exhibit increased ankle instability 6 months after their injury than athletes who did not suffer a lateral ankle sprain

Though such a title is quite inclusive and a relatively complete sentence, the sentence itself is 29 words and 182 characters (with spaces) long—much longer than most journals would allow for a title. Paring down the extraneous words, one could easily generate a functional title such as:

Increased ankle instability exists in athletes up to 6 months after an inversion ankle sprain

and an even more honed version could be written as:

Prolonged ankle instability exists in athletes after an inversion sprain

Though this last example is lacking relevant details, it illustrates just how much editing can be done to a "complete" title while still communicating the manuscript's main intent. From the original title, this abridged version is now just 10 words and 72 characters. Though it is arguably a sentence fragment, it remains grammatically correct to a good degree and communicates the main purpose of the study. A reader whose interest in lateral ankle sprains in athletes has been piqued by this article title could then be expected to examine the abstract or even full text to obtain additional information.

Humor in Titles

Similarly, humor in a title is generally frowned upon as it can bias the reader into thinking that the quality of the article is diminished.[8] Consider the following:

Increased skeletal muscle force production after an acute anxiety-inducing event: Evidence that we are all a little Incredible Hulk-like inside

Though this title puts a humorous twist in referencing a classic superhero, this would only be relevant to those familiar with American comic books or 1980s television. Those unfamiliar with the comic book legend may end up scouring the article to figure out just what the "Incredible Hulk" is and how it influenced the experiment. Likely, manuscript authors will not have a description or brief history of the Hulk in the manuscript, instead relying on what may be a false assumption that the article readers will be familiar with the Hulk. Those readers unfamiliar with the Hulk would likely spend additional time trying to orient themselves as to what this ultimately unnecessary part of the title is referring.

Acronyms and Abbreviations in Titles

Abbreviations or acronyms are generally frowned upon in a manuscript title. Even common abbreviations such as CPR or MRI—which are almost certain to be understood by a journal's readership—should be written out as "cardiopulmonary resuscitation" and "magnetic resonance imaging," respectively. The rare exception might be abbreviations associated with measurements (eg, MHz, cm), equipment model numbers, or professional associations (eg, APTA, CAATE). However, the journal's *Author's Guide* may have specific allowances for other abbreviations or acronyms.

Drafting an Effective Title

Many authors start out with a manuscript title in mind as soon as drafting of the manuscript begins. While early drafting of the title is logical, it is not generally recommended in the event that the direction of the manuscript changes over time. Therefore, authors are better off waiting until the final stages of manuscript writing to develop a title. Furthermore, developing a manuscript

Sidebar 7-1

Assuming an interested researcher reads a title at a speed of 5 words per second, a title limited to a 16-word maximum must market the entire article to that researcher in just over 3 seconds.

title near the final stages of the manuscript process ensures that the manuscript context is more defined and the overall scope of the manuscript is likely better established. These aspects can then be captured more effectively in a well-written title.

Prior to writing the title, the overall purpose of the manuscript (ie, the aim or aims) as well as the study results should be established, as each will likely be conveyed through the title. This can be somewhat challenging, as it calls for condensing the message originally discussed throughout 20 to 30 pages of double-spaced text down to 1 short fragmented sentence (Sidebar 7-1).

Shorter titles are generally recommended,[2] but the evidence of whether longer titles help or hurt an article's citation likelihood is somewhat conflicting.[9,10] To maximize the effect of the title and keep it as condensed as possible, authors should strive for a happy medium between titles that are too long and too short by ensuring that every word in the title has meaning. Much like what was discussed in Chapter 3 regarding selection of the right word(s), title word or character limitations set out by a journal require that any words that do not contribute to the message of the title should be removed.

Investing time in crafting a well-written manuscript title can have important dividends for the author. Appropriate titles can contribute to a favorable perception of the article, convince the reader to invest in reading the abstract and main text of the article, and influence web search results, which can ultimately increase the article's citation count. Therefore, it is important during the manuscript development process for authors to set aside ample time to develop an effective and inclusive title.

The Abstract

If the title is the most-read component of an article, the abstract is the runner-up. "Informative" manuscript abstracts (as compared to indicative abstracts associated with books, essays, etc) are often included along with the title in web search results, and a manuscript's abstract is typically published in conference proceedings. Abstracts are designed to provide the reader a summary of the most pertinent information in an article in a format that allows the abstract to stand alone from the main text. The word abstract itself is derived from *ab* ("from") and *trahere* ("to draw"), indicating that the very purpose of the abstract is to "draw out" pertinent information, in this case from the article. While the article title draws the reader in, the abstract sells the article by providing a more detailed overview of the article's content. Perusing a well-written abstract allows the reader to know why the study was conducted (ie, what gap existed in the literature), what the study found, and what can be learned from the study's results. While the article's title must grab the reader's attention, the abstract should serve to provide an overview of the article in a way that makes the reader want to access the complete article.

As often occurs with the title, abstracts are bound by the word limit constraints set out by each journal's *Author's Guide* (see Chapter 6 for more information). Typical word limits for manuscript abstracts average around 200 to 300 words, and abstracts that do not reach the full word count limit are acceptable. Because of the word limit, each section (eg, introduction, methods) of the manuscript that is summarized in the abstract should not expect to exceed 2 to 3 sentences. It is also important to remember that even though the abstract is part of the manuscript, and should be

Sidebar 7-2

You might compare drafting the manuscript title and abstract to operating a business. In doing so, think of the main manuscript as your company store. The title would therefore be equivalent to the company sign—it is out for everyone to see, it sums up your business in 3 to 5 words, and it likely has a bit of a "catchy" aspect to it to draw the attention of potential customers amid all of the other signs around it. Similarly, your abstract would serve as the advertisement flyer. It shows what your business is involved with, it highlights the most important items, and it is designed to get people inside your store. People who find an item they are interested in might then enter the store (ie, read the full manuscript) but after holding or seeing the item up close ultimately decide that it is not for them. Others drawn in by your sign and/or flyer may ultimately purchase the item, which could be considered the equivalent of a citation.

Sidebar 7-3

There are generally 2 types of abstracts—those that summarize a main manuscript text and those that function as an individual representation (ie, without an associated manuscript). Conference abstracts are generally the type submitted independent of a manuscript, and as such are required to stand alone and convey all relevant information without the assistance of the manuscript to "fill in the holes." Because of the lack of an associated manuscript, conference abstracts will often (but not always) allow a higher word count than journal abstracts. Because they are independent submissions, conference abstracts typically deviate from "full manuscript abstract" rules in that they may contain required acronyms, include references, etc.

written in the same style as the manuscript, it is at the same time a stand-alone section. Therefore, an abstract should not be constructed by cutting-and-pasting sentences from the manuscript body. This approach of abstract development will lead to a rather disjointed and choppy abstract flow.

Because the abstract is summarizing the manuscript, it is imperative that all material found in the abstract is also contained in the manuscript body. The reader has the expectation that what is read in the abstract will be described in more detail in the full text; therefore, failing to include the abstract's information in the full manuscript will leave the reader uninformed and possibly questioning the validity of the information (Sidebar 7-2).

Like the manuscript title, the abstract is usually drafted after the manuscript body has been finalized. Drafting an abstract prior to writing the manuscript will fail to account for manuscript revisions, ultimately requiring a subsequent revision of the abstract as well. When drafting each section of the manuscript (eg, introduction, methods), the author should extract the most relevant information essential to the manuscript and use that information in the abstract. For example, sample size (n), participant demographics, or study limitations are not generally included in an abstract as the information is not vital to understanding what the study was about or what was found. If, however, a reader wanted more information about these aspects after reading the abstract, he or she should be able to find the additional details in the main article (Sidebar 7-3).

Author's Guide instructions for many journals will often outline the sections required for abstracts, while other journals have no specific format for the abstract outside of the word limit. The main manuscript body will then likely follow the same structure as the associated abstract headings in most cases. In general, abstracts utilizing a traditional IMRaD format will follow a relatively consistent pattern:

- Introduce the topic and state the problem or knowledge gap that exists (~2 sentences)
- State how or why the current study will fix the problem or knowledge gap (1 sentence)
- Outline the study design, participants/subjects pool, and general methodology (1 sentence)
- List general demographics, findings, and relevant statistics (optional) (~2 sentences)
- Elaborate on what the findings represent as well as conclusions of the study (~2 sentences)

As an example of what should be included in the abstract but elaborated on in the manuscript text, consider the following abstract excerpt:

> *A randomized control design was utilized to evaluate the effects of ultrasound with passive stretching compared to ultrasound alone for the reduction of delayed-onset muscle soreness in college-aged male and female participants.*

This one excerpt provides information regarding the study design, participant characteristics, and study purpose, all highly relevant information for the study. The number of subjects as well as the ultrasound settings are not vital to the message conveyed in the abstract and as such are not included, though they will certainly be required for the methods and results section of the full manuscript. As written, an individual interested in understanding whether nonsteroidal anti-inflammatory drugs (NSAIDs) influence muscle pain might be intrigued by this abstract enough to look in the main article text to see if NSAID users were excluded from the study. Those inclusion and exclusion criteria are not relevant information for the abstract, but as any reviewer would agree, these criteria are essential for the full manuscript.

Writing Tense

By the time a manuscript abstract is written, it is likely that the author has already submitted an outline of the research project to their institution's review board, and they have likely submitted a grant proposal which in all probability required an abstract or summary of the project. It would be easy to simply use one of those previously submitted abstracts as the basis for the manuscript abstract as the general focus of the research as well, since the methodology has likely changed little. However, the writing tense of both a review board abstract as well as a grant proposal abstract are written in future tense as they outline what the researcher will do. Conversely, manuscript abstracts detail research that has already occurred. Therefore, past tense writing is required for abstracts. For example, a grant abstract may state:

> *Participants will then complete 3 sets of 10 repetitions of seated leg extensions at 75% of their 1RM.*

Written for a manuscript abstract, this same activity would need to be changed to:

> *Participants completed 3 sets of 10 repetitions of seated leg extensions at 75% of their 1RM.*

Though it is a small change, it is important to ensure that the abstract reflects that the research has already been conducted. To save valuable writing time, portions of a grant or review board abstract may be incorporated into the relevant sections of the subsequent manuscript abstract. If so, the author must dedicate ample time revising the methods and writing tense to reflect that the research has already occurred.

Tips to Limit the Abstract Word Count

Because journals set a word count limit for abstracts, it is imperative that the author approach writing an abstract similar to how he or she writes a title and minimizes the use of extraneous words. For example, authors should work to avoid unnecessary use of words such as "which" and "that," words that when used in a particular way contribute little to the manuscript and ultimately increase the word count. For example:

Analysis revealed that the experimental group's mean score did not change significantly after exercise, which indicated that the intervention was ineffective.

loses no meaning by simply removing the extraneous words "which" and "that":

Analysis revealed the experimental group's mean score did not change significantly after exercise, indicating the intervention was ineffective.

When possible, minimize or avoid the use of acronyms in the abstract. It is not always possible to completely avoid acronym use in the abstract; however, using acronyms will require the author to spell out the words associated with each acronym the first time they are used. This will further increase the abstract's word count for each acronym used. Whereas the main manuscript does not always have a word count limit, placing the acronym (and associated spelling out of the acronym) in the manuscript body rather than the abstract will free up additional text opportunity in the abstract.

As discussed briefly earlier, details regarding methodology as well as statistical analysis are often withheld from the abstract. Because the main manuscript body will detail the methodology, nothing more than a general sweeping statement about study methods is required for an abstract. Researchers interested in details regarding the methods used will direct themselves to the main text if necessary. Statistics will be outlined in the results section, but when included in an abstract are typically limited to the probability value, such as:

Results indicated a significant dosage effect (P < .05) on strength, vertical jump height, and power, but no significant difference for time.

For manuscript abstracts, citations should not be placed in the abstract (individual/conference abstracts will require citations and associated references). Because everything discussed in the abstract must be mentioned in the manuscript text as well, the more comprehensive and elaborative main manuscript text would better facilitate the use of citations compared to the more concise requirement of the abstract.

Conclusion

Proficiency in title and abstract writing are essential for a quality manuscript. Being the most visible portion of an article, a well-crafted title should catch the reader's attention and make him or her want to read the abstract to understand the context of the article. The abstract should then be written in a way that encourages the reader to read the main text. This in turn disseminates the information found in the associated research study, hopefully either stimulating future research or impacting medical practice. Because of the impact that a quality title and abstract can have, manuscript authors should reserve ample time to ensure that both the title and abstract adequately convey the message carried in the manuscript.

References

1. Fox CW, Burns CS. The relationship between manuscript title structure and success: editorial decisions and citation performance for an ecological journal. *Ecology and Evolution.* 2015;5(10):1970-1980.
2. Mack CA. How to write a good scientific paper: title, abstract, and keywords. *Journal of Micro/Nanolithography, MEMS, and MOEMS.* 2012;11(2):020101.
3. Akman T. Selection of authors, titles and writing a manuscript abstract. *Turk J Urol.* 2013;39(Suppl 1):5.
4. Soler V. Writing titles in science: an exploratory study. *English for Specific Purposes.* 2007;26(1):90-102.
5. Day R. *Write and Publish a Scientific Paper.* 4th ed. Cambridge, England: Cambridge University Press; 1994.
6. Hyland K. What do they mean? Questions in academic writing. *Text.* 2002;22(4):529-558.
7. Aleixandre-Benavent R, Montalt-Resurecció V, Valderrama-Zurián JC. A descriptive study of inaccuracy in article titles on bibliometrics published in biomedical journals. *Scientometrics.* 2014;101(1):781-791.
8. Armstrong JS. Readability and prestige in scientific journals. *Journal of Information Science.* 1989;15(2):123-125.
9. Habibzadeh F, Yadollahie M. Are shorter article titles more attractive for citations? Crosssectional study of 22 scientific journals. *Croat Med J.* 2010;51(2):165-170.
10. Jamali HR, Nikzad M. Article title type and its relation with the number of downloads and citations. *Scientometrics.* 2011;88(2):653-661.

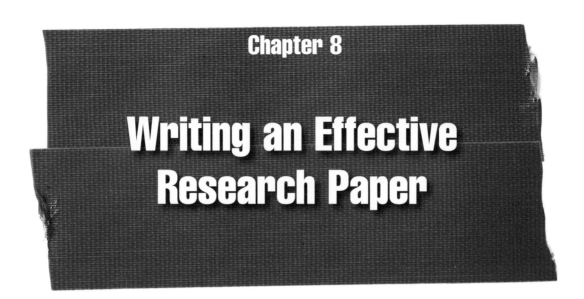

Chapter 8

Writing an Effective Research Paper

Craig R. Denegar, PhD, PT, ATC, FNATA and
Jay Hertel, PhD, ATC, FACSM, FNATA

Why write a research manuscript? Perhaps the question is better phrased: why does one want or need to write?

- To share knowledge and shape the future
- To fulfill responsibilities as a clinician, educator, or scholar
- To graduate
- Future employment or salary depend on it
- All of the above

Depending on the stage of one's life as a student, health care provider, researcher, or educator any or all options may be "correct." Whether altruistic or self-preserving, writing is a professional responsibility that for most is ultimately rewarding, but not easy. In fact, writing is hard, often frustrating work. As outlined in Chapter 1, writing unveils one's ideas, beliefs, knowledge, and ability to convey thoughts, ideas, and concepts through words. Ultimately, writing is a permanent record for all to read, critique, and offer comment. Whether a high school term paper "enriched" through the use of copious amounts of red ink, or the harsh comments from a reviewer about a paper submitted for publication, most authors have asked themselves, "Why do I put myself through this?"

The answer to that question likely varies among authors, but most do it because it is intrinsically, and sometimes extrinsically, rewarding. For a manuscript author, reading that the product of his or her labor in conducting and reporting research has been accepted for publication—and knowing the work will be a permanent addition to the body of science—is always cause for celebration. The moment of acceptance, when a manuscript becomes an article, erases all the angst, anger, and frustration experienced leading up to success. Many an author has quietly expressed that he or she will never write another book, review, or research paper again, only to return to the grind in search of that intrinsic reward of being viewed as a scholar.

Knoblauch M. *Professional Writing in Kinesiology and Sports Medicine* (pp 77-88).
© 2019 Taylor & Francis Group.

Authors experience all the emotions associated with writing across the spectrum of research reports to books. Writing is work. Practice, and growing through the review process, can build efficiency and lighten the perceived burden. This chapter reflects our evolution as authors and is divided into both a discussion of overarching strategies for effective writing and a section of more granular suggestions for writing each portion of a manuscript. It is hoped that this chapter will lighten the load for manuscript authors and make the writing experience more efficient and enjoyable.

Strategies

Writing effectively requires organization, patience, and practice. The intent of this chapter is to help develop effective research manuscript writing strategies. According to the reporter and humorist Franklin P. Jones, "Experience is that marvelous thing that enables you to recognize a mistake when you make it again."[1] The insight provided within this chapter would not be possible without the learning that occurred through mistakes made and the thoughtful criticism received from editors and reviewers.

Many of the mistakes made by novice writers are the result of poor conceptualization and organization of the desired research manuscript. These writers began at the beginning, hoping to find the end point. Sometimes the path forward becomes obvious, sometimes it is rather convoluted, and there are many beginnings still hanging out there, never having found an end. Begin writing with an outline and use it (see Chapter 2 for an overview of drafting an effective outline). A well-crafted outline provides order of the primary themes and concepts and connects the sections into a coherent story. This chapter was built on an outline. The text fills in the gaps. A failure to build an effective outline often leads to writing more than is needed to convey the purpose, detail the methods used to collect data, report results, and discuss the findings in the context of science and clinical practice. The challenge of the lack of a complete outline and the use of far too many words is often encountered when working with students. When mentoring students, a paper may shrink by 25% after careful editing yet improve markedly.

A research report is typically organized with an Introduction, a Methods section, the Reporting of Results, and a Closing Discussion (ie, the IMRaD format) that leads the reader to a conclusion that answers, or at least adds insight about, the question posed in the introduction.[2] An abstract of the work (see Chapter 7) precedes the main text but is typically the last element to be written. Authors typically write a research manuscript section by section. It is easy to lose sight of the big picture. The reader should be provided with a cohesive story that connects the reason for doing the work and questions asked, the methods used to collect the data, what was observed, and finally how the results align with existing knowledge. In clinical research, the Discussion section should also inform the reader as to the clinical and practical applications of the findings. Once a complete draft of the work has been completed, consider whether a reader will follow the logic of the author(s) from the introduction to the conclusion. This may be best accomplished by asking a colleague to read the work and by auditing the organization of the paper against the outline of the paper.

Once an outline has been developed and the actual writing process has begun, strive to use plain language. President Bill Clinton issued a Memorandum on Plain Language in Government Writing in an effort to make government documents more easily understood by the citizens of the United States. Scientists and scholars often complain that their work is not appreciated or fully understood. Similarly, manuscript authors must also ensure that they do not lose the message in the words. To reduce the chance of this happening, authors should strive to write in a manner that makes the work understandable to a broad audience. Research related to health care should

Table 8-1. Valuable Resources for Authors to Consult When Writing a Research Manuscript

RESOURCE	FOCUS	WEBSITE
CONSORT Statement	CONsolidated Standards of Reporting Trials	www.consort-statement.org
STARD Statement	Standards for Reporting of Diagnostic Accuracy	www.stard-statement.org
STROBE Statement	STrengthening the Reporting of OBservational studies in Epidemiology	www.strobe-statement.org
PRISMA Statement	Preferred Reporting Items of Systematic reviews and Meta-Analyses	www.prisma-statement.org
PEDro Scale	Physiotherapy Evidence Database methodological quality scale	https://www.pedro.org.au/english/downloads/pedro-scale
QUADAS-2 Scale	QUAlity of Diagnostic Accuracy Studies scale	www.bristol.ac.uk/population-health-sciences/projects/quadas/quadas-2

be described in a manner that a "typical" patient can understand. If a colleague only peripherally knowledgeable about the work cannot understand the article's purpose or results, it is likely most consumers will also struggle, and ultimately put the paper aside.

Few are born prepared for scientific writing, and the preparation of a research manuscript is not particularly creative. The early experience and preparation of most people who become writers is in a creative vein, meaning that they are allowed to develop their writing in a method that works best for them. Remember second grade? The first assignment of the year was a 500-word essay about summer vacation. After 350 words the important information has been delivered about the trip to (fill in the blank); a great story had been told, only to have it ruined by the need to find 150 more words to complete the assignment. Authors may be limited in the number of words permitted by a journal but rarely, if ever, expected to reach a word count. Readers appreciate the concise delivery of the information sought.[3]

There are a number of useful tools that are designed to ensure that authors include all of the critical components of content in a research manuscript. These tools include, but are not limited to, the CONSORT checklist for randomized controlled clinical trials, the STARD statement for diagnostic studies, the STROBE checklist for observational studies, and the PRISMA checklist for systematic reviews and meta-analyses. Using one of these appropriate tools during the writing process serves to make writing easier while providing the reader a very clear understanding of the research process. The use of tools intended for the research consumer such as the QUADAS-2 checklist and the PEDro scale can also be very useful in writing. These instruments identify gaps in the information provided and help the author recognize limitations that warrant discussion later in the manuscript. The links to these documents can be found in Table 8-1. Lastly, students and novice authors tend to rush to submit, relieved that the work is done. It is better to write, set the paper aside for a few days, revisit and edit, share with a colleague or two, revise, and then submit for review. The additional time spent in this process will be returned in responding to reviewer comments. Editors and reviewers strive to improve a manuscript, and it is humbling to a manuscript author when easily identified flaws are pointed out by reviewers.

Manuscript Sections

Introduction

The introduction to a research manuscript should build toward the main purpose or purposes of the research and thus the manuscript. A useful exercise is to read all of an introduction section except the purpose statement and then try to predict the purpose. In a well-written introduction, the purpose of the study should be strikingly obvious when it is revealed.

The following issues should be concisely addressed in the introduction:

- What is the big picture, clinical, or scientific problem?
- What is known about the problem?
- What is not known about the problem?
- How will filling in the knowledge gap help solve the problem?
- What is the purpose of the current study?
- What are the research hypotheses?

A well-written introduction can be thought of as a funnel. A funnel is broadest at the top, which could parallel the description of the overarching problem that outlines the direction of the manuscript's purpose. For example, when performing health sciences research, the "big picture" problem is often the societal burden of a particular pathology. The societal burden is often described in the context of epidemiology (How many people are affected by the pathology?) or severity (What are the typical outcomes in patients with the pathology?) of the pathology being studied. Previous literature should be referenced liberally throughout the introduction.

As the introduction progresses, the funnel begins to narrow as the author explains what is known and unknown about a few specific aspects of the pathology. Using the example above, in a study aiming to examine the etiology of a particular pathology, the author will likely describe what is known and unknown about the causes for developing the pathology. Alternatively, in a study addressing treatment interventions, the author might describe what is known and unknown about specific treatments for the given pathology.

As the funnel continues to narrow, the manuscript author then must linearly lead the reader from what is unknown about the topic to the purpose of the manuscript by informing the reader how the current study will fill the identified knowledge gap and help improve the scientific understanding or clinical management of the problem.

The purpose statement(s) and research hypothesis represent the bottom of the funnel. If a manuscript addresses multiple aims, they should be delineated into primary and secondary categories. Each stated purpose should then be followed with a research hypothesis that is directional (eg, greater, have more, weigh less) in nature (as opposed to a null hypothesis indicating no difference).

With any big picture problem, there are many important research questions that could be asked and answered; however, a well-written research manuscript will focus on only a single, or certainly no more than a few, specific research question. A common error of novice researchers is to try to answer too many research questions or address too many purposes in a single study (Table 8-2).

Table 8-2. Differences Between a Research Question and a Purpose Statement

	GOAL	STRUCTURE	EXAMPLE
PURPOSE STATEMENT	Tell the reader the overall aim of the research study.	Declarative statement where the sentence ends with a period (.)	The purpose of the study was to compare the effectiveness of lace-up and semi-rigid ankle braces in the prevention of ankle sprains in high school basketball players.
RESEARCH QUESTION	Tell the reader what specific question the study is designed to answer in an effort to achieve the purpose statement.	Query ending in a question mark (?)	Are lace-up or semi-rigid ankle braces more effective at preventing ankle sprains in high school basketball players?
RESEARCH HYPOTHESIS	Tell the reader the expected answer to the research question at the outset of the study.	Directional statement of the expected results of the study.	Our hypothesis was that semi-rigid ankle braces would be more effective than lace-up braces at preventing ankle sprains in high school athletes.

Methods

The Methods section should be written at a level of detail that allows an informed reader to be able to replicate the study methods. As such, the methods portion of a manuscript must clearly describe the research design, study participants, instruments, procedures, data processing, and statistical analysis used in the study. The writing of the methods should allow the article's reader to easily follow the methodology used to acquire the data reported in the Results section.

Many authors choose to use the first paragraph of the Methods section to provide a roadmap for the rest of the Methods section. Some authors refer to this as the *design paragraph* because it typically includes a description of the specific research design used, as well as identifying the independent and dependent variables in the study. The description of research design is usually made with universally accepted experimental design terms that describe the structure of study such as randomized controlled trial, prospective cohort study, or case-control study (please note that this is not an exhaustive list of study design terms). Many journal author guidelines provide guidance on desired terminology to be used in specific journals. When listing independent variables, authors should be sure to list the specific levels of each independent variable to make it clear to the reader what comparisons will be made. For example, in a study comparing the effects of 2 treatments over 3 time points, the following description would be used: the independent variables were treatment group (experimental, sham) and time (baseline, immediately post-treatment, 2 weeks post-treatment). The dependent variables, or outcome measures, should also be clearly described and, if relevant, be delineated as primary and secondary outcomes to align with the purpose statement.

While describing the study design, it is essential for authors to describe procedural details such as allocation, randomization, and blinding that are critical to the appraisal of the methodological quality of a study by an informed reader. A CONSORT flow chart is recommended to concisely illustrate the design and flow of participants through the study design (Figure 8-1).

There is considerable variation in the literature as to how research study participants are described. The most common descriptors are patients, participants, volunteers, or subjects, although less generic terms such as students or astronauts can be used if they are more

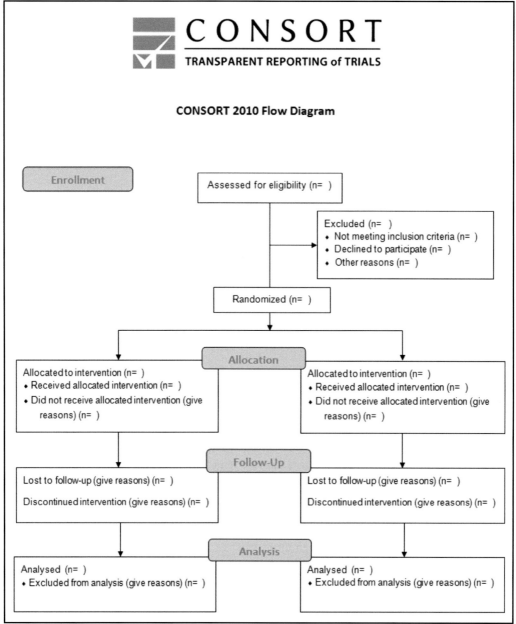

Figure 8-1. A CONSORT flow chart illustrates the flow of study participants throughout the course of a research study. Readers are able to see how many participants took part, or dropped out, at each step of the study. (Reprinted with permission from The CONSORT Flow Diagram. CONSORT Web site. http://www.consort-statement.org/consort-statement/flow-diagram. Accessed September 26, 2018.)

representative. Whichever term an author chooses to use, that term should be used consistently rather than interchanging multiple terms (eg, student, participant, patient). In addition, the number of participants should be provided along with important demographic information to help the reader contextualize who was studied. Relevant demographic information often includes details of the sex, age, and anthropometric measures (height, body mass, body mass index, etc) of participants, but should also include other information relevant to health status. For example, in a study of patients with knee osteoarthritis, it would be appropriate to indicate the average

Table 8-3. Sample Demographic Table

DEMOGRAPHICS (MEAN ± SD)

CHARACTERISTIC	CHRONIC ANKLE INSTABILITY	CONTROL
Paticipants	15	15
Sex (M/F)	5/10	5/10
Age (y)	23 ± 4.2	22.9 ± 3.4
Height (cm)	173 ± 10.8	173 ± 9.4
Mass (kg)	72.4 ± 14	70.8 ± 18
No. of previous sprains	4.5 ± 3.2	N/A
Godin score	94 ± 47	84 ± 40
FAAM ADL	87.2 ± 7.1	100
FAAM Sport	68.5 ± 5.7	100

SD = standard deviation; FAAM = Foot and Ankle Ability Measures; ADL = activities of daily living; N/A = not applicable

Reprinted with permission from Kautzky K, Feger MA, Hart JM, Hertel J. Surface electromyography variability measures during walking: effects of chronic ankle instability and prophylactic bracing. *Athletic Training & Sports Health Care.* 2015;7:14-22.

Kellgren-Lawrence scale grade of participants. Patient demographics are typically presented in a table to provide an efficient overview of the characteristics of each group of participants (Table 8-3). In addition, the recruitment strategy for the study should also be detailed so the reader can easily ascertain how participants became aware of the study prior to enrollment. Likewise, the inclusion and exclusion criteria for study participation and the screening procedures to ascertain these criteria should also be described.

It is important to explicitly indicate that both: (1) study participants provided informed consent to participate in the research study (or indicate why this was not necessary), and (2) the study methods were approved by an appropriate research ethics board. Many journals also require authors to indicate the registration of clinical trials with an appropriate agency such as www.clinicaltrials.gov.

A paragraph describing the technical instruments used in the study typically appears next. In this paragraph, the make, model, and manufacturer of each important instrument is described. However, it is important that the manuscript author limit this section to a description of the equipment only; outline what equipment was used, but refrain from venturing into the study procedures (ie, how the equipment was used). In addition to physical pieces of equipment (eg, machines, tools), it is also common for authors to describe what survey instruments, such as patient-reported outcome or screening tools, were used.

The meat (apologies to vegetarians) of the Methods section is the description of the study procedures. A thorough description of how the outcome measures (dependent variables) were taken and how the interventions (independent variables) were applied is required. Here, the manuscript author should outline a chronological description of what occurred once subjects were enrolled in the study. If baseline measures were taken, begin by describing how each measure was taken. Conversely, if only post-intervention measures were taken, describe the procedures of the interventions first and then the measures. If previously published procedures were used, be sure to cite these references appropriately. Use figures and tables to help succinctly describe how the measures and interventions were applied. For example, if a study used an agility test as an outcome measure, it may be easier to use a computer-generated figure or series of photographs to describe how the agility test was performed rather than trying to explain it in several sentences of text. Likewise, if an exercise progression was used as an intervention, it may be easier to detail the progressions in a table or figure rather than in text. Because the manuscript author is often intimately familiar with the study methods, it may be easy to assume that readers will have the same level of familiarity. This assumption is flawed, so authors must be sure to provide the technical details of the procedures at a level of detail that allows others to replicate the study methods.

In studies that involve more than simple data manipulation (ie, taking an average score from 3 trial repetitions) to determine an outcome measure, it is common to have a paragraph or two that detail data processing procedures. This is especially common when data are recorded using a digital signal. For example, if surface electromyography is used to assess the electrical activity of skeletal muscle contractions during walking, there are many steps of data manipulation prior to the calculation of the value that will be used as a participant's score for statistical analysis. In this case, the author would need to detail how the electromyographic signal was amplified, filtered, rectified, and smoothed before calculation of a peak (or other relevant) value. Reporting the order that these data manipulations occurred is critical as are the mathematical or technical details of each step. While reading this level of detail may be mind-numbing to some readers, the author should strive to convey this essential information in a manner that is accessible and understandable to informed readers, and allows for a smooth flow of how data were handled prior to analysis.

The final part of the Methods section should be a description of the statistical analysis. The independent and dependent variables should be reiterated and followed by a thorough description of the statistical procedures that were performed. Primary, as well as follow-up (post hoc), analyses should be described at a level of detail to allow for replication of the analyses. These should include all inferential analyses (*t* tests, ANOVA, etc) and magnitude-based comparisons (effect sizes, confidence intervals, etc) that were performed. Most importantly, if an analysis is reported in the Results section, it should be described in the Statistical Analysis section. Likewise, if an a priori *P* value was established, it should be listed. It is also recommended that an a priori sample size estimate (sometimes called a "power" analysis) be included in this section as well.

Results

The Results section of the research manuscript can be likened to the box score detailing the outcomes of a baseball game. The box score will tell you the results of the game (the home team won 3 to 2, which players got hits, how many strikeouts each pitcher recorded, etc), but it will not tell you why these results occurred or why they are important in a broader context (the home team moved into a tie for first place with this victory!). This latter information would be described in a text-based newspaper story about the game's results but would not be detailed in the box score. Similarly, the Results section of a manuscript should be thought of as "just the facts"; therefore, in the case of reporting research, those facts are represented as quantitative data obtained as outlined in the Methods section. What the data (ie, study results) mean in the bigger picture (as described in the opening sentence or two of the Introduction section) will be described in the Discussion section immediately following the Results section.

Results should be reported in the order of priority established in the introduction. If the data are insufficient to draw conclusions regarding the primary question, this should be the first finding reported, or on occasion, the introduction revised so that the most important finding can be reported first. Reordering can become problematic, however, as the introduction must build the case for asking the primary question.

The use of plain language is particularly important when reporting results. The reader should learn about what was observed, not the statistics. For studies evaluating group comparisons, emphasize the direction (which group had higher or lower scores than the other?) and magnitude (how much higher or lower were the scores?) of differences, rather than the results of the inferential statistical tests. Consider a study where stretching of the gastrocnemius/soleus complex was compared to joint mobilization for the restoration of dorsiflexion range of motion following an acute lateral ankle sprain, and accept the assumption that greater improvement was observed following joint mobilization.

Which statement best conveys the finding?

An independent t *test revealed significant between-group differences* (t(25) = 7.6, P = .023), (Mean stretching = 4.5 +/- 2.4°, Mean mobilization 6.8 +/- 2.2°).

Or

We observed greater improvement in dorsiflexion range of motion following joint mobilization (6.8 +/- 2.2°) than stretching (4.5 +/- 2.4°) ((t)25) = 7.6, P = .023).

The first sentence is about the results of the statistical test, while the second sentence is about which treatment produced the better result and uses that statistical result to contextualize the differences found. If there is doubt as to whether what the investigators observed is clearly conveyed, ask a student or a colleague in clinical practice. Practicing clinicians in particular are interested in what was observed and have little use for the statistic.

It is good practice to use tables and figures effectively when presenting the results. The adage "a picture is worth 1000 words" holds true in scientific writing. The author should consider the best means of presenting the results prior to beginning to write the Results section. Will specific findings be best reported in the manuscript text, a table, a figure, or some combination of these? As the investigator, the manuscript author is well-versed as to the nature of the data, has extensively read research reports, and can anticipate how the report will be constructed. Authors are encouraged to think creatively about the presentation of results.[4] For example, does a simple bar or line graph that shows group means provide the best representation of the results? Or, would the graphing of the pre-post change scores of individual participants provide a more robust illustration of the study results? Alternatively, if there are multiple dependent variables in a study, are these best conveyed to a reader in a table or in multiple univariate graphs? Or, could all of the variables be visualized on a single image such as a radar graph?

Manuscript authors should also consider the structure of tables and figures before the data are analyzed. When tables and figures are developed in the final rush to finish a paper, it becomes more likely that one or more reviewers will suggest better options for conveying the results. While these misjudgments were not fatal, such mistakes cost time in terms of revising the manuscript or could ultimately lead to a rejection that might have been avoided with planning and preparation.

Another important principle is to avoid redundancy between information conveyed in figures, tables, and text. The same quantitative results should only appear in one of these 3 places as page space is at a premium in quality peer-reviewed journals.

Discussion

The Discussion section is where the author contextualizes the results of the study into the existing knowledge on the topic. This section follows the order established in the introduction and carried through the methods and results to allow the reader to follow the story from start to finish. The first paragraph of the discussion should clearly articulate whether the research hypotheses were confirmed or refuted. The primary results should be discussed first, not a robust discussion of a secondary finding. Although the content of a Discussion section will depend on the specific results a study, the basic outline of the Discussion section can be developed once the methods are established. Outlining the Discussion section early may prevent the writing of a long—and not particularly informative—section that fails to lead the reader straightforwardly to the key findings and conclusion of the research project.

The Discussion section should not be viewed as an opportunity to simply reiterate the results without having to report those pesky statistics. Instead, authors are encouraged to begin the

Discussion section by indicating whether their research hypotheses were confirmed or refuted. This should be followed by a nuanced description about why the study's results most likely occurred and what the broader implications of those results are (remember the box score vs newspaper analogy from the previous section). Identifying what the research study's new findings add to the literature and how the study's results compare to what is already known is paramount to a well-written discussion. This is even more important if the results were unexpected and may require a rethinking of existing theory, dogma, or accepted paradigms.

A common error manuscript writers often make is to try to explain away unexpected results by indicating that the original methods used must have been flawed. For example, if a study assessing the efficacy of therapeutic ultrasound failed to result in the hypothesized improvement in patient outcomes, the author may be tempted to develop a list of reasons why the hypothesized results were not found. These might include potential reasons like the incorrect patients were recruited into the study or the wrong ultrasound parameters were prescribed. The author may be tempted to conclude that if these "errors" were corrected the research hypothesis would have been confirmed, but they should refrain from this. If a precise research question is asked and a robust study design is executed to answer that question, the answer to the question is important whether the research hypothesis is confirmed or refuted. If researchers already knew the answer to the research question, there would be no need to do the study. While unexpected results can initially be disconcerting, it is important for authors to brainstorm for all possible explanations of the results and not quickly jump to the conclusion that "we must have done the experiment wrong."

All studies have limitations, and authors should be forthright in acknowledging the limitations of their study in the latter half of the Discussion section. Inexperienced authors may think that if they do not mention their study limitations, peer reviewers might fail to recognize them. Experienced authors will do the exact opposite with the thought that it is better to criticize one's self than to be criticized. By acknowledging a study limitation up front, the author is in control of the issue rather than the reviewer. The concept of writing about study limitations is addressed in more detail in Chapter 10.

When delimitations exist, the experienced author will often indicate why he or she made the choice that he or she did by writing about the potential weaknesses of alternative approaches. These issues often involve a balance of internal validity and external validity. Internal validity involves the robustness of the study design, while external validity represents the generalizability of the results to situations outside of the completed study. A decision to increase the internal validity of the study (eg, limiting the inclusion criteria to only the most severely impaired patients with a particular pathology) would provide greater experimental control, but it would limit the external validity of the study because the results could not be generalized to patients with less severe impairments. Authors should always be cautious about overgeneralizing the importance and application of their results.

Most Discussion sections end with a single concluding paragraph. This paragraph should concisely reiterate the most important findings and applications of the study. Inexperienced authors are often tempted to conclude that "further research is needed"; yet, however true this statement may be, it should not be the conclusion of a research manuscript. More research will always need to be done—on all topics, in all disciplines, forever. Concluding that more research is needed diminishes the findings of the study described in the manuscript. The conclusions should clearly answer the research questions posed in the introduction. The principles of writing strong conclusions are elaborated on in Chapter 10.

References

A reference or citation identifies a source of information. A reference serves 2 important yet different purposes. First, a reference acknowledges the contributions of other authors to the body of knowledge. A reference also directs the reader to previous work on a subject so that he or she

Sidebar 8-1

Searching for a paper for which the reference was inaccurate is time consuming and frustrating. In the days before computer software, large numbers of references were incorrect. The consumer was left to comb a library to find a paper for which the author or volume, issue, or page numbers were not accurately communicated, not knowing which piece of information was in error.

can gather more information and consider the application of results in the context of his or her research or practice.

The failure to acknowledge the work or ideas of someone else and thus intentionally, or unintentionally, have them appear as one's own is plagiarism. Plagiarism and the related topic of copyright infringement are discussed in detail in Chapter 14. Acknowledging the contributions of others is only a part of an author's responsibility.

It is important to recognize that references are important to readers. Rarely do clinicians and scientists read a paper in an area of interest and not seek more information in one or more references. This process has become considerably easier in the digital age as many articles available online now have direct links embedded within the reference.

Citing the work of others is not difficult, however, much like the preparation of other aspects of the manuscript, the author must consult the style requirements of the journal (see Chapter 6) to which a paper is to be submitted. The most common format for citing references in medical journals is that prescribed by the American Medical Association.[5] However, other disciplines, and some health care journals, use the style prescribed by the American Psychological Association.[6] The style prescribed by the Modern Language Association[7] is yet another set of guidelines to appropriately reference the work of others.

Lastly, after having formatted the references in accordance to the prescribed style, manuscript authors should verify that the reference list is accurate. Correctly formatted and accurate references save a lot of time and effort on the part of copyeditors. The use of software such as RefWorks (ProQuest LLC) makes the job of formatting and accurately citing the work of others much easier. The use of such software is highly recommended. Copyeditors continue to find the need to check references, and often claim that while the number of incorrect references has decreased, the problem has not been eradicated (Sidebar 8-1).

Title and Abstract

It could be argued that the most important components of a research manuscript are the title and abstract. These topics are discussed in detail in Chapter 7. Recognize that many readers only decide to read an entire paper after scanning a title and abstract to gauge the extent to which the paper addresses their needs and interest. Thus, careful attention should be devoted to crafting the title and abstract after the body of the manuscript is completed. The title and abstract are not add-ons, but rather the sales pitch for your work.

Submitting the Manuscript

The manuscript should not be submitted for review until all of the authors have had the opportunity to read the entire manuscript and are satisfied with the title, abstract, body of the manuscript, and all figures and tables. While manuscript submission can be anticlimactic (it still needs to get accepted for publication!), it is hoped that this overview of writing the traditional research manuscript has provided a set of useful guiding principles for getting to this point in the publication process. Just as proper foresight and planning are essential to designing a quality research study, these same attributes are requisites for writing a quality research manuscript.

References

1. Jones FP. *Brainy Quote*. https://www.brainyquote.com/quotes/quotes/f/franklinp121323.html. Accessed June 15, 2018.
2. Knight KL, Ingersoll CD. Structure of a scholarly manuscript: 66 tips for what goes where. *J Athl Train*. 1996;31(3):201-206.
3. Knight KL, Ingersoll CD. Optimizing scholarly communication: 30 tips for writing clearly. *J Athl Train*. 1996;31(3):209-213.
4. Weissgerber TL, Milic NM, Winham SJ, Garovic VD. Beyond bar and line graphs: time for a new data presentation paradigm. *PLoS Biol*. 2015;13(4):e1002128. doi: 10.1371/journal.pbio.1002128.
5. *AMA Manual of Style: A Guide for Authors and Editors*. 10th ed. Oxford, England: Oxford University Press; 2007.
6. VandenBos GR, ed. *Publication Manual of the American Psychological Association*. 6th ed. Washington, DC: American Psychological Association; 2010.
7. *MLA Handbook*. 8th ed. New York, NY: Modern Language Association of America; 2016.

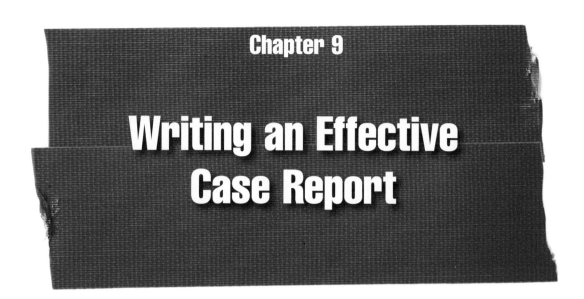

Chapter 9

Writing an Effective Case Report

Laura Kunkel, EdD, LAT, ATC, PES

Always note and record the unusual … Publish it. Place it on permanent record as a short, concise note. Such communications are always of value.[1]
—Sir William Osler, father of modern medicine

What Is a Case Report?

Case reports describe a patient with a particular condition or who underwent a particular procedure or a situation that occurred in a particular clinical environment. For example, the diagnosis and treatment of a patient with a rare injury or disease could be described or one who was treated with a new treatment or surgical procedure. An example of a case report regarding a situation in a particular clinical environment might be one that explains a general approach taken to the management of care for an athlete with unique needs (eg, anterior cruciate ligament deficient, sickle cell trait). The design of a case report is descriptive and may be prospective or retrospective. Prospective studies examine an event forward in time, while retrospective studies look back at a case that has already occurred. Descriptive research studies aim to describe a variable or phenomenon of interest. There is not usually a hypothesis or manipulation of variables, and no correlational or cause and effect relationships are established. However, the Discussion portion of a case study may compare the results with others published in the literature (Sidebars 9-1 and 9-2).[2-4]

Traditionally there are 2 types of case reports: diagnostic-related and management-related.[5] Diagnostic-related case reports are exploratory in nature, such as when a relatively unique or rare condition is encountered. Developing a case report allows the author to explore the condition further through the literature and offers the reader the opportunity to learn about a condition he or she might not otherwise be aware of. Unique findings are reported in diagnostic case reports as a means to educate clinicians about alternate or irregular presentations of either common or uncommon conditions. An example of a need for a diagnostic case report might include a particular

Knoblauch M. *Professional Writing in Kinesiology and Sports Medicine* (pp 89-98).
© 2019 Taylor & Francis Group.

Sidebar 9-1

Case reports are often referred to as *case studies*; however, most sports medicine journals use the term *case report*, therefore, in this chapter we will use this term. You should understand that both terms are referring to case reports.

Sidebar 9-2

A *case series* is similar to a case report; however, a group of patients is studied, rather than just one or a few.[2-4]

condition that is rare in overall health care, or perhaps a condition that is relatively common in health care (eg, pregnancy) but rare in a specific population (eg, swimmers).[6] In some cases, diagnostic-related case reports can also focus on rare comorbidities, such as a clotting disorder or neurological disease that might be missed or misdiagnosed.[7]

Management-related case reports can be used to apply external evidence in a real-world setting. For example, management-related case reports could be used to investigate the effectiveness of an intervention recommended by a particular systematic review, meta-analysis, or clinical practice guideline. The management-related case report can outline how well the recommended intervention worked in a setting with a particular patient population.[8] Management-related case reports may also be exploratory. For example, a management-related case report might discuss a unique intervention that shows promise or outline a new or rare side effect associated with that intervention.[5,7] For examples of situations that have warranted the development of a case report, see Table 9-1.

It is often thought that only those cases in which the patient outcome was positive hold valuable information for practicing clinicians and researchers. In fact, some journals favor acceptance of case reports in which positive outcomes were found, although clinicians can learn from both positive and negative outcomes.[9] Just as in medical debriefing, it is important for practitioners to learn from mistakes or negative outcomes. Examples of mistakes or negative outcomes that might be included in a case report include no-fault errors and adverse events. A no-fault error is an error that occurred because the practicing clinician did not have the knowledge needed to make an appropriate clinical decision.[8] Adverse event reports, in which a potentially causal relationship between a medical product or treatment and an adverse event is suspected, can identify possible problems and stimulate further investigation.[10] Therefore, reports in which the patient outcome was negative can also serve as a valued source of evidence. Despite unfavorable outcomes, other researchers and clinicians can learn from case reports with negative outcomes in the same way they can learn from case reports with positive patient outcomes (Sidebar 9-3).[11]

Case reports have a relatively low ranking in the hierarchy of evidence[12]; however, they are still valuable forms of research for the practicing clinician. Case reports allow detection of new conditions, discovery of different approaches to treating common conditions, and formation of hypotheses, which can then be tested with further research. Many higher levels of evidence such as randomized controlled trials were conducted after a published case report sparked initial interest in the subject. It is this initial curiosity that can lead medicine to further advance. For example, the first publications regarding AIDS back in 1981 were case series reports.[13,14] The first human heart transplant was also documented by case report.[15] In fact, of 103 case reports and case series published in *The Lancet* from January 1996 to June 1997, 23 (22.3%) were followed by randomized controlled trials (Sidebar 9-4 and Figure 9-1).[16-20]

Table 9-1. Case Report Examples

Uncommon condition	Wang WL, Mares A. Bilateral epidural hematoma with parietal skull fracture in a division I college athlete: a case report. *J Sport Rehabil.* 2017;26(5):415-417.
	A Division I football player suffered a bilateral epidural hematoma and parietal skull fracture from falling down a flight of stairs.
Common condition with a unique presentation	Murray SR, Reeder MT, Compton MR. Weighted-ball training leading to a stress fracture of the distal ulna in a collegiate softball pitcher. *Athletic Training & Sports Health Care.* 2017;9(3):138-140.
	A collegiate softball player suffered a distal ulna stress fracture caused by 4 weeks of training with a weighted ball.
Common condition, but uncommon in athletes	Shaffer JD. Recovery from a posterior hip dislocation: a case report. *Int J Athl Ther Train.* 2016;21(3):19-23.
	A 16-year-old football player returned to play just 3 weeks after dislocating his right hip.
Rare comorbidities	Casmus RJ, Paider B, Messick B, Guy JA. Iliotibial band rupture associated with an acute knee dislocation in a collegiate football player. *Athletic Training & Sports Health Care.* 2017;9(5):233-237.
	A self-reducing knee dislocation in an 18-year-old football player is described. Resulting trauma included complete ruptures of the ACL, PCL, LCL, posterior lateral corner, and iliotibial band as well as partial tearing of both heads of the gastrocnemius, vastus medialis and lateralis, biceps femoris, and semimembranosus.
Unique intervention	Oglesby LW, Gallucci AR. Medial patellofemoral ligament double avulsion in a collegiate American football athlete: a case report. *Int J Athl Ther Train.* 2017;22(3):52-56.
	The rehabilitation of an 18-year-old football player with a double avulsion of the MPFL is discussed. No known literature existed describing rehabilitation of MPFL multiple avulsion repair.
Rare side effect	Loopike MF, Winters M, Moen MH. Atrophy and depigmentation after pretibial corticosteroid injection for medial tibial stress syndrome: two case reports. *J Sport Rehabil.* 2016;25(4):380-381.
	Two cases of women with medial tibial stress syndrome who experienced atrophy and depigmentation of the skin after pretibial corticosteroid injections are presented.

ACL = anterior cruciate ligament; LCL = lateral collateral ligament; MPFL = medial patellofemoral ligament; PCL = posterior cruciate ligament.

Sidebar 9-3

Reid, Kremen, and Oppenheim provide one example of a case report in which the patient outcome was unfavorable, published in *Sports Health*.[11] The authors describe a 13-year-old male soccer player who suffered a traumatic popliteal artery occlusion. Orthopedic evaluation was delayed, and the patient suffered from lower extremity ischemic necrosis, septic pulmonary thromboembolism, systemic shock, and death. The authors were able to use the negative outcomes of the case to outline the importance of immediate and careful vascular examination after closed knee injuries in young athletes.

Sidebar 9-4

Hierarchies, or levels of evidence, allow us to rate the quality of evidence in order to determine its usefulness. The type and quality of evidence determines where it falls in the hierarchy, and clinicians should strive to utilize the highest level available to solve their clinical problem. Although case reports fall fairly low in the hierarchy, often they are the highest level of evidence available about a certain topic. For example, sometimes rare disorders do not have enough patients with the condition to warrant a randomized controlled trial; therefore, our clinical question and subsequent literature search might lead us to only case reports. Levels of evidence were first described by the Canadian Task Force on the Periodic Health Examination in 1979,[17] and have been expanded upon and modified by others over the years.[18,19] Sackett, Haynes, and Tugwell created the evidence pyramid in 1985,[20] often used or modified by organizations and authors still today. A more contemporary evidence pyramid is shown in Figure 9-1.[18]

Figure 9-1. Evidence pyramid showing the hierarchy of evidence.[18] Case reports are quite valuable in bridging communication between practicing clinicians and academic researchers. One way this occurs is when a clinician publishes or presents a case report and a researcher becomes interested in the condition or treatment of interest, then conducts a higher-level study to learn more. In addition, clinicians can report on clinical outcomes or events with real patients rather than laboratory-based subjects. Information about clinical situations regarding actual patient outcomes is very valuable in contributing to a profession's body of knowledge.[7]

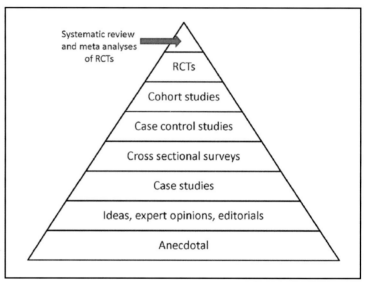

Case reports have their limitations as well. In general, findings from case reports cannot be generalized to the population due to the low sample size of one or only a few patients and the lack of randomization or manipulation of variables. In addition, patient confidentiality cannot be fully guaranteed; however, all efforts should be made by the author to maintain confidentiality. Authors must refrain from using patient or school names, naming specific places such as a medical facility, or using dates that may reveal protected patient information. Finally, causality cannot be inferred because there is no manipulation or control of variables, and case reports typically do not give the reader new statistical data about a condition. However, as stated above, case reports are sometimes more feasible than randomized controlled trials and can lead to more robust exploration of conditions. Therefore, case reports are valuable sources of evidence.

Before Getting Started

There are a few considerations that need to be made prior to writing a case report. First, the author is responsible for obtaining consent from the patient/subject. Some journals offer example consent forms to help authors develop their own. In addition, regulations set forth by the Health Insurance Portability and Accountability Act of 1996 (HIPAA) must be adhered to. All patient identifying information should be removed when writing a case report. Every effort needs to be made to ensure patient privacy.

In addition, authors should consult their Institutional Review Board (IRB) regarding whether approval is needed for the project. Case reports do not meet the US Department of Health and Human Services definition of research, which is "a systematic investigation, including research development, testing and evaluation, designed to develop or contribute to generalizable knowledge,"[21] because the project is not methologically driven and data are not analyzed. Therefore, these projects do not typically need to be approved by an IRB; however, some IRBs hold policies that exceed the US Department of Health and Human Services requirements and authors should check with their IRB for specific policies.

Writing a Case Report

Before writing a case report, it is important to first establish which journal the authors intend to send the case report to, and then refer to that journal's *Author's Guide* for case report formatting requirements (see Chapter 6). Typically, sports medicine journals require 3 major sections of a case report: Introduction, Case, and Conclusions and/or Discussion. In general, the content of these sections remains relatively consistent between journals. Next, each of these sections is outlined in more detail.

Introduction

The Introduction of a case report serves to describe the clinical problem,[22] giving an overview of the condition of interest. This overview should include available evidence from the literature regarding what is currently known, such as the etiology or epidemiology of the condition as well as characteristics related to the diagnosis, prognosis, or therapy. One might incorporate how common the condition is in a given population, common risk factors, or how the condition is diagnosed.[23] The Introduction should not contain rudimentary information that the anticipated audience would be expected to know, such as the anatomy or basic physiology of the body area. Information unnecessary for a full understanding of the case and condition of interest is also to be avoided (eg, whether a bacteria is gram-positive or gram-negative). In some journals, a clear description of how the case report will potentially make a meaningful contribution to the literature is also included in this section.[23] Overall, the Introduction should serve to build an argument for the importance of the case report. See Sidebar 9-5 to practice identifying relevant and irrelevant material in the Introduction of a case report.

Case

Sports medicine journals typically require a body, which presents the case report to the reader. The patient, intervention, comparison, and outcome (ie, PICO)[24] technique can be used as a guide for writing this section of the case report.[23] First, a thorough description of the patient (or in some cases, setting, if the case report covers issues such as a bacterial outbreak) should be outlined. It is essential that relevant patient characteristics (ie, age, sex, activity or occupation) are outlined to provide the reader a thorough framework of the case. The chief complaint, patient history, and physical exam should be included as well.[3,22-24] Specific to patient history, authors should be sure to include a history of the patient's condition, including symptoms and relevant events leading the patient to seek advanced care.[23]

> ## Sidebar 9-5
>
> An estimated 80,000 to more than 250,000 ACL injuries occur each year, with more than 50% occurring in athletes 15 to 25 years old. The ACL functions to control joint motion by stabilizing the tibia on the femur. It originates from the lateral femoral condyle and inserts into the intercondylar notch and various portions are taut throughout the range of motion. While ACL injuries are common in sports that require quick changes of direction, they are relatively rare in distance running.

To this point in the case report everything has likely been subjective in nature. Next, the reader should be provided details that are more objective, requiring interaction with the medical professional. For example, physical examination and evaluation findings, range of motion or muscle testing results, imaging and/or lab findings, and the final diagnosis should be included.[3,22-24] There is no required minimum or maximum amount of details; rather, it is up to the author to decide what information contributes to providing an adequate background of the patient or event that the case report is centered around.

Much like any published journal article, the case report serves to expand the current knowledge of medicine. In other words, the case report should function to provide medicine-related information that is of benefit to others. Up to this point in the drafting of the case report, no real benefit to the reader has been provided (except perhaps in those cases where a diagnosis of a rare condition has been outlined) as nothing has been reported specific to how the case was managed. However, the next section of a case report serves to inform the reader as to what was done (ie, treatment) for the subject of the case report, providing the treatment protocol or case management, including a detailed account of the interventions used,[3,22,24] clinical course[3] and timeline of when outcomes were assessed,[23] and final outcome of the case.[22,24] Criteria for return to activity should also be discussed.[3] This provides the reader with an overview of the handling of the case and whether the intervention was successful based on measureable outcomes. In the event that a clinician reading the case report has a similar patient or event (as determined by information in the background and presentation sections), he or she can compare the treatment and outcomes to determine if a similar course of action might be successful with his or her particular patient. If the outcomes were not favorable in the case report, it still provides the clinician important information as he or she could choose an alternate treatment.

Conclusions and/or Discussion

Conclusions and Discussion are outlined at the end of the case report. Some journals, such as *Sports Health*,[11] require both sections while others, such as the *Journal of Athletic Training*,[3] combine these into one section. Here, the case report author should present a relevant analysis of the uniqueness of the case report,[3,22,23] referencing existing literature. The unusual presentation, characteristics, or treatment of the patient should be highlighted with an overall statement of why the case report is unique or rare compared to other already-existing literature.[23] The clinical implications—or how the case can impact clinical medicine—as well as discussion of its importance to other health care providers should also be discussed.[22,23] However, because case reports lack a high level of scientific rigor, the writer should avoid sweeping generalizations to other patients and cause-and-effect statements. Finally, the author should close the case report with recommendations for future research, particularly research that is directly initiated by the case report findings (Sidebar 9-6).[23]

Sidebar 9-6

Case reports are warranted when a unique or rare condition or clinical situation is presented; however, what makes something unique or rare? *Unique* can be defined as the atypical presentation of key features in the case, as compared to previous literature. *Rare* can be defined as conditions that are rare in a population and potentially threatens life or limb.[8]

General Tips for Writing a Case Report

Novice writers often make similar mistakes when writing case reports. Because case reports often highlight particular patients or events rather than a detailed experiment inherent to a randomized controlled trial, the writing of a case report requires a particular style. Students in kinesiology and/or sports medicine often have their first foray into scientific writing by way of the case report, and in so doing it is often that similar errors appear in the writing. Therefore, in addition to the information regarding scientific writing provided in Section I of this book, here are a few recommendations on addressing various mistakes commonly seen in case report drafts, along with examples.

Using Dates

When describing the timeline of the clinical course, use number of days, weeks, or months rather than dates. Using a particular day, say August 4th, 2017 tends to "date" the case report and reveal its age. Imagine, for example, a researcher finds a case report that matches his or her patient. Despite matching her patient's situation well, in the treatment section, the clinician reads "the patient first visited the physician in April of 1974." Once seeing the actual date, the clinician may feel that the case report is outdated as it was written more than 40 years ago, even though the preferred treatment is still in use today. In addition, the US Department of Health and Human Services Office for Human Research Protections advises against using dates to ensure de-identification of patient information.[25] Dates can be used, but should be limited to rare situations and only when necessary to provide essential information regarding the case report, such as "The flu outbreak of 2016 was among the worst on record." Specific to using dates, another example follows:

> *Incorrect: A female basketball player complained of right ankle pain, which began on January 4, 2017. Upon physician examination, radiographs and MRI were ordered. On January 11, 2017 results were obtained that indicated a syndesmosis ankle sprain as well as a distal fibular fracture. An open reduction with internal fixation was performed on January 25, 2017.*

> *Correct: A female basketball player complained of right ankle pain. Upon physician examination, radiographs and MRI were ordered. Results were obtained 1 week later and indicated a syndesmosis ankle sprain as well as a distal fibular fracture. An open reduction with internal fixation was performed 3 weeks after the initial examination.*

Using Abbreviations

Many journals offer a list of acceptable abbreviations that can be used without definitions. Be sure to note these and use them accordingly per each journal's requirements outlined in the *Author's Guide*, and define any abbreviations not found on the journal's list. In addition, it is not recommended that authors create their own abbreviations or use those unique to a particular clinic. All abbreviations used should be commonplace in clinical medicine.

Incorrect: ORIF was performed 3 weeks after the initial examination.

Correct: An open reduction with internal fixation (ORIF) was performed 3 weeks after the initial examination.

Use Past Tense When Describing Your Patient Case

Because the events happened in the past, use past tense when describing the patient case. Any information about current clinical practice or evidence could be described in present tense.

Incorrect: A female basketball player complains of right ankle pain. Upon physician examination, radiographs and MRI are ordered. Results are obtained 1 week later and indicate a syndesmosis ankle sprain as well as a distal fibular fracture. An open reduction with internal fixation is performed 3 weeks after the initial examination.

Correct: A female basketball player complained of right ankle pain. Upon physician examination, radiographs and MRI were ordered. Results were obtained 1 week later and indicated a syndesmosis ankle sprain as well as a distal fibular fracture. An open reduction with internal fixation was performed 3 weeks after the initial examination.

Always Write in the Third Person

Don't use terms such as "we" or "I." Instead, use "the health care provider," for example.

Incorrect: We performed soft tissue release and joint mobilization techniques to address the loss of joint range of motion.

Correct: Soft tissue release and joint mobilization techniques were performed to address the loss of joint range of motion.

Use Contemporary Terminology

Avoid the use of slang that is often used in the day-to-day work of a health care provider (ie, "rehabilitation," rather than "rehab" or "emergency department" or "trauma center" rather than "emergency room"). In addition, be sure to use current contemporary terminology, as indicated by major professional organizations (ie, "athletic trainer" rather than "trainer").

Incorrect: Upon release from the ER and physician follow-up, the patient began a rehab program.

Correct: Upon release from the emergency department and physician follow-up, the patient began a rehabilitation program.

Write in Complete Sentences

Avoid the more condensed method of writing patient notes. Remember the case report is not an outline of patient notes, rather it is scientific writing.

Incorrect: Patient reported to the athletic training clinic complaining of right knee pain.

Correct: The patient reported to the athletic training clinic complaining of right knee pain.

Conclusion

Case reports are a valuable source of evidence to enhance clinical practice and, if clearly written, provide the reader with valuable medical insight from the clinical medicine setting. In addition, the cost of conducting a case report is low compared to that of more formal research studies. Time to publication is also typically faster, and case reports can be used to explore problems that could not be studied with experimental research due to ethical constraints.[9] For example, a clinician might find a valuable case report explaining how an adverse reaction to iontophoresis was managed in a patient, however, ethical limitations would not allow a researcher to conduct a randomized controlled trial by purposely subjecting participants to an adverse reaction to iontophoresis. Through well-written case reports, health care can be enhanced by learning from the experiences of others and further robust research may be conducted based on the ideas expressed in them.

References

1. Thayer WS. Osler, the teacher. *Bulletin of the Johns Hopkins Hospital*. 1919:51-54. https://archive.org/stream/sirwilliamoslerb00bloguoft/sirwilliamoslerb00bloguoft_djvu.txt. Accessed August 14, 2017.
2. Manuscript submission guidelines. *Am J Sports Med*. www.sagepub.com/sites/default/files/upm-binaries/82010_AJSM426265_SubmissionGuidelines.pdf. Accessed August 13, 2017.
3. Author's guide. *J Athl Train*. 2010. https://jat.msubmit.net/html/2010%20Authors'%20Guide.pdf. Accessed August 13, 2017.
4. Manuscript submission guidelines. *Orthop J Sports Med*. 2017. journals.sagepub.com/pb-assets/cmscontent/OJS/OJSM_Manuscript_Submission_Guidelines_July_2017.pdf. Accessed August 13, 2017.
5. Haq RU, Dhammi IK. Effective medical writing: how to write a case report which editors would publish. *Indian J Orthop*. 2017;51(3):237-239.
6. Medina-McKeon JM, McKeon PO. Horses and unicorns and zebras, oh my! a model for unique versus rare case studies. *Int J Athl Ther Train*. 2015;20(3):1-3.
7. McKeon PO, Medina McKeon JM. Case studies: the alpha and omega of evidence-based practice. *Int J Athl Ther Train*. 2014;19(6):1-3.
8. Medina-McKeon JM, King MA, McKeon PO. Clinical contributions to the available sources of evidence (CASE) reports: executive summary. *J Athl Train*. 2016;51(7):581-585.
9. Nissen T, Wynn R. The clinical case report: a review of its merits and limitations. *BMC Res Notes*. 2014;7:264.
10. Kelly WN, Arellano FM, Barnes J, et al. Guidelines for submitting adverse event reports for publication. *Drug Saf*. 2007;30(5):367-373.
11. Reid JJ, Kremen TJ, Oppenheim WL. Death after closed adolescent knee injury and popliteal artery occlusion: a case report and clinical review. *Sports Health*. 2013;5(6):558-561.
12. Sackett DL. Rules of evidence and clinical recommendations on the use of antithrombotic agents. *Chest*. 1989;95(2 Suppl):2S-4S.
13. Gottlieb MS, Schanker HM, Fan PT, Saxon A, Weisman JD. Pneumocystis pneumonia: Los Angeles. *Morbidity and Mortality Weekly Report*. https://www.cdc.gov/mmwr/preview/mmwrhtml/june_5.htm. Published June 5, 1981. Accessed August 14, 2017.
14. Gottlieb MS, Schroff R, Schanker HM, et al. Pneumocystis carinii pneumonia and mucosal candidiasis in previously healthy homosexual men: evidence of a new acquired cellular immunodefinciency. *N Engl J Med*. 1981;305(24):1425-31.
15. Kantrowitz A, Haller JD, Joos H, Cerruti MM, Carstensen HE. Transplantation of the heart in an infant and an adult. *Am J Cardiol*. 1968;22(6):782-790.
16. Albrecht J, Meves A, Bigby M. Case reports and case series from Lancet had significant impact on medical literature. *J Clin Epidemiol*. 2005;58:1227-1232.
17. Canadian Task Force on the Periodic Health Examination. The periodic health examination. *Can Med Assoc J*. 1979;121(9);1193-1254.
18. Sackett DL. *Evidence-Based Medicine. How to Practice and Teach EBM*. New York, NY: Churchill Livingstone Inc; 2000.
19. OCEBM Levels of Evidence Working Group. *The Oxford 2011 levels of evidence*. http://www.cebm.net/ocebm-levels-of-evidence. Accessed August 14, 2017.
20. Sackett DL, Haynes RB, Tugwell P. *Clinical Epidemiology: A Basic Science for Clinical Medicine*. Boston, MA: Little, Brown; 1985.

21. Office for Human Research Protections. Code of federal regulations, title 45 part 46. *US Department of Health and Human Services web site*. https://www.hhs.gov/ohrp/regulations-and-policy/regulations/45-cfr-46/index. html#46.102. Published January 15, 2009. Accessed November 25, 2017.
22. Information for authors. *Med Sci Sports Exerc*. http://edmgr.ovid.com/msse/accounts/ifauth.htm. Accessed October 12, 2017.
23. Guidelines for authors: CASE reports. *Int J Athl Ther Train*. http://journals.humankinetics.com/page/authors/ijatt.
24. Instructions to authors. *J Orthop Sports Phys Ther*. 2017;1-6. http://www.jospt.org/page/authors. Accessed October 12, 2017.
25. *Summary Table of Recommendations on the HIPAA Privacy Rule*. hhs.gov. https://www.hhs.gov/ohrp/sachrp-committee/recommendations/2004-september-27-letter-summary/index.html. Updated July 10, 2017. Accessed February 7, 2018.

Chapter 10

Matching Your Writing to the Individual Section of the Research Paper

Rehal Bhojani, MD, FAAFP, CAQSM

Overview of IMRaD Traditional Sections

As stated in previous chapters, there are 4 traditional sections in a journal manuscript,[1,2] each of which outlines a specific component of the research:

1. Introduction (Why was the study undertaken? What is the research question and hypothesis?)
2. Methods (How was the study conducted?)
3. Results (What data were found with respect to the research question?)
4. Discussion (What do the results imply toward the research question? Perspectives for future research?)

These sections are the current standard in form and style, which was born in England and France nearly 300 years ago in a peer-review process.[3] This structure has been tested and validated for centuries and allows readers to easily navigate an article to find relevant and pertinent material. Over time, as the fields of research and medicine have expanded and become more robust, it has been argued that the IMRaD format has become too restrictive as it often does not correlate well with the sequence of events required for research. As far back as 1964, Nobel laureate Peter Medawar criticized this shortcoming specific to the IMRaD format of a scientific paper in his oration "Is the scientific paper a fraud?":

> I do not mean that the interpretations you find in a scientific paper are wrong or deliberately mistaken. I mean the scientific paper may be a fraud because it misrepresents the processes of thought that accompanied or gave rise to the work that is described in the paper ... The scientific paper in its orthodox form does embody a totally mistaken conception, even a travesty, of the nature of scientific thought.[4]

Whereas Medawar was critical of a scientific paper not embracing the flow of scientific thought, it has also been pointed out that the restrictive nature of the IMRaD format may not allow for

Knoblauch M. *Professional Writing in Kinesiology and Sports Medicine* (pp 99-109).
© 2019 Taylor & Francis Group.

clarifying specific points made in the 4 main IMRaD sections. In a subsequent corollary to the Medawar paper, Howitt and Wilson added:

> There is, of course, a good reason why the scientific paper is highly formalized and structured. Its purpose is to communicate a finding and it is important to do this as clearly as possible. Even if the actual process of discovery had been messy, a good paper presents a logical argument, provides supporting evidence, and comes to a conclusion. The reader usually does not need or want to know about false starts, failed experiments, and changes of direction.

> This approach to scientific communication has implications for teaching undergraduates the nature and practice of science as it creates a completely wrong impression of how science actually works and perpetuates a stereotype of scientists as logical and rational beings, doggedly adhering to the scientific method. Students may confuse the presentation of a logical argument with an accurate representation of what was actually done. This leads to a view of science that is unrealistic and may even be damaging as it implies that failure, serendipity, and unexpected results are not a normal part of research.[5]

Scientific papers are meant to convey findings in a concise manner; however, as studies have evolved, the ability to articulate these findings in the IMRaD structure may be more difficult at times. The creation of additional headers can help circumvent some of the traditional section limitations. Specifically, the International Committee of Medical Journal Editors (ICMJE) commented on the importance of subsections within a manuscript:

> Long articles may need subheadings within some sections (especially Results and Discussion) to clarify their content. Other types of articles, such as case reports, reviews, and editorials, probably need to be formatted differently.[6]

Because of its long-standing use, the IMRaD format is typically referenced when discussing the drafting of a research manuscript. With the increased prevalence of journals requiring subsections, however, there has been little guidance or strategy on what to write or how to write these subsections, as well as how to avoid repetition between a subsection and its main section (eg, Discussion).

Overview of New Subsections in the Literature

In recent years, subsections have begun to emerge in various journals to highlight a particular aspect of a research study. Some journals require these new subsections as part of a manuscript submission whereas other journals merely recommend various subsections. A clear understanding of what the expectations are for these subsections with regards to content, writing style, and specifications will allow the author to maximize his or her manuscript's impact.

Review of Various Sports Medicine Journal Requirements

There are a variety of subsection requirements across journals in the kinesiology and sports medicine field. A sampling of these subsections is listed in Table 10-1.

Introduction to New Subsections

As discussed, almost all journals require the IMRaD format for original research manuscripts. Specific to subsections, however, there is no consistent set of required subsections (eg, Conclusion, Limitations) between journals. Nevertheless, manuscript authors will find that certain subsections

Table 10-1. Sports Medicine Journal Subsections as Noted in Manuscript Preparation	
JOURNAL	**OTHER SUBSECTION HEADINGS (IN ADDITION TO THE IMRAD)**
The American Journal of Sports Medicine	• Conclusion • Clinical Relevance • Key Terms • Study Design • Background
British Journal of Sports Medicine	• Conclusion • Clinical Relevance
Sports Medicine	• Acknowledgments
Journal of Bone and Joint Surgery	• Conclusion • Source of Funding
Clinical Orthopaedics and Related Research	• No additional subsections
Medicine & Science in Sports & Exercise	• Conclusion
Exercise and Sport Sciences Review	• Conclusion/Summary • Perspectives
International Journal of Sports Physiology and Performance	• Conclusion • Practical Applications
Journal of Science and Medicine in Sport	• Conclusion • Practical Applications
Journal of the American Academy of Orthopaedic Surgeons	• No additional subsections
Journal of Athletic Training/Athletic Training Education Journal	• No additional subsections
International Journal of Sports Medicine	• Acknowledgments
Journal of Sports Sciences	• No additional subsections
European Journal of Sport Science	• No additional subsections
Physical Therapy in Sport	• Conclusion
Clinical Journal of Sport Medicine	• No additional subsections
ACSM's Health & Fitness Journal	• No additional subsections
Gait & Posture	• No additional subsections
International Journal of Athletic Therapy and Training	• No additional subsections
Journal of Orthopaedic & Sports Physical Therapy	• Key Points

are commonly encountered across multiple journals, which highlights the importance of following each journal's *Author's Guide* (see Chapter 6) to format the manuscript correctly. Because of the frequency by which these common subsections are encountered, an overview of several of these subsections will be provided next.

Conclusion Subsection

Arguably, one of the most common subsections in a journal article is the Conclusion subsection. The Conclusion subsection is typically inserted at the end of the Discussion, yet serves to offer a slightly different perspective than the Discussion section itself. Whereas the discussion provides a summary as well as relevance of the research project, the embedded Conclusion subsection affords an opportunity for the manuscript author to summarize the discussion and briefly outline the work performed in the study. More specifically, it "should commensurate with the design used and results obtained ... (and) should not go beyond the limits of the study conducted."[7] This section should be clear by using simple language that leaves no confusion, concise in addressing only the issues outlined in the manuscript, and objective through avoiding inferences and vague statements.

In a series of articles written on manuscript preparation, Angel Borja offers a simplistic overview of the general purpose of the Conclusion subsection, stating " ... [t]his section shows how the work advances the field from the present state of knowledge." He further goes on to state that manuscript authors should " ... provide a clear scientific justification for your work in this section."[8(p13)]

Despite Borja's view of the Conclusion, medical journals have differing recommendations with regard to the Conclusion subsection. For example, *The American Journal of Sports Medicine* submission guidelines direct manuscript writers to " ... [s]tate the answer to your original question or hypothesis. Summarize the most important conclusions that can be directly drawn from your study."[9(p1)] Journals with a more specific focus outline the conclusion differently. For example, the *Journal of Bone and Joint Surgery* submission guidelines state that " ... [t]he conclusion should include: major factors limiting the longevity of the prosthesis at the time of this follow-up; recommendations regarding the continued use of the prostheses if it is still available; if the prostheses is not still available, lessons applicable to the current successor or to similar designs."[10(p2)] Because variation exists even within the Conclusion subsection between journals, it is vital that manuscript authors tailor their conclusion to match the requirements of the particular journal to which he or she is submitting. The Conclusion subsection with respect to content should have the following[11-13]:

- Remind the reader of the research problem and purpose and how each was addressed
- Briefly summarize what has been covered in the paper
- Make some kind of holistic assessment/judgment/claim that pertains to the whole project (ie, more than a descriptive summary)
- Assess the value/relevance/implications of the key findings in light of existing studies and literature
- "Speak" to the Introduction
- Outline implications of the study (for theory, practice, further research)
- Comment on the findings that failed to support or only partially support the hypothesis or research questions directing the study
- Refer to the limitation(s) of the studies that may affect the validity or the generalizability of results
- Make recommendations for further research
- Make claims for new knowledge/contribution to knowledge

Although the requirements of the Conclusion subsection are often outlined in the *Author's Guide* of the journal, the style in which the Conclusion subsection is written is generally left up to the manuscript author. Specific to writing style, it is important that manuscript writers be cognizant of the journal's type of readership when writing the Conclusion subsection. The conclusion provides the reader with the focus of what the research discovered. Therefore, manuscript authors should review their results with the literature and use the new knowledge as the focus of their conclusion. The style of the Conclusion subsection can also be based on the type of manuscript and location of the section. In original articles, as discussed above in *The American Journal of Sports Medicine* and *Journal of Bone and Joint Surgery* examples, there are specific recommendations regarding what the journal editors' desire in a Conclusion subsection. In review articles as well as perspective articles, the Conclusion subsection will typically focus more on the limitations of current knowledge and the future direction of research.

Writing an effective Conclusion subsection takes practice, but a well-written conclusion serves the difficult job of taking the data and discussion findings and outlining the importance of the manuscript in the overall scope of a particular field.

> *Effective protection against VF [ventricular fibrillation] with chest wall protection of modest thickness can be achieved in an animal model of commotio cordis. It is reasonable to expect that chest protector designs incorporating these novel materials will be effective in the prevention of commotio cordis on the playing field.*[14(p30)]

Note a few stylistic points in this example. First, each sentence presents one idea instead of multiple, which helps ensure that there is no repetition of ideas in this short subsection. Furthermore, the language is easy to read and not composed of technical jargon. The purpose of the paper, along with a holistic claim, is presented concisely. Finally, there are no grand claims in this subsection; rather, the author simply infers that based upon findings from the study's research, the novel materials should be expected to prevent commotio cordis. Here is another example:

> *Surgical treatment of primary acute patellar dislocation leads to significantly lower rate of redislocation and provides better short-medium clinical outcomes; whereas in the long-term follow-up, results of patients treated conservatively were as good as those of surgical patients. Unfortunately, the overall quality of the body of evidence is low. Further randomized controlled trials, describing anatomical abnormalities and soft-tissue integrity that may influence the choice of treatment, are needed.*[15(p521)]

In this conclusion, note how the authors clearly identified the shortcomings (lack of quality of body of evidence in the literature) as well as future ideas (randomized controlled trials for treatment) for research. The shortcomings could also be written as a limitation (discussed shortly). If a reader were to glance at this subsection of the article first, it would give a concise objective answer to the question posed in the hypothesis. Using the earlier example, writing it in another way illustrates how quickly the conclusion loses its overall impact:

> *Surgical treatment of primary acute patellar dislocation leads to significantly lower rates of redislocation and provides better short-medium clinical outcomes. The long-term follow-up, results of patients treated conservatively, were as good as those of surgical patients. The overall quality of the body of evidence is low. Randomized controlled trials describing anatomical abnormalities and soft tissue integrity that may influence the choice of treatment are needed.*

Note that the removal of certain words and sentence structure reduces the impact of the conclusion in general.

If there is a Conclusion subsection requirement in the Abstract, the limited used of words allowed in the abstract requires that the focus of the conclusion should be on the implications and the "bang" statement. As discussed in Chapter 7, readers will regularly scan an abstract first to see if the article is relevant to their topic of interest. Specifically, readers will often migrate to the Conclusion subsection first to determine the relevance of the study and thereby determine if the article is worthwhile. A well-crafted conclusion statement in the abstract can help engage the reader's interest in the full article.

Conclusion Versus Perspectives

In some journals, such as the *Exercise and Sport Sciences Review*, Perspectives or Future Perspectives replaces the Conclusion subsection. Depending on the article type, sometimes "perspectives" is a more appropriate heading to the section (especially review articles) as this subsection may draw out other types of ideas in a more reflective manner. As an example, the paragraph below was part of a Conclusion and Perspectives subsection:

> *Exercise-induced increases in MPS [muscle protein synthesis] are longer lived and peak later in the UT [untrained] state than in the T [trained] state, resulting in greater overall MPS, and likely greater net protein accretion, in the UT state. This observation indicates that RT [resistance training] must adaptively induce changes in processes that modulate MPS, but these currently remain elusive. The responses of MyoPS [myofibrillar protein synthesis] are even harder to predict, as there is a paucity of data; however, the available evidence indicates that the increases after RE point to responses that are qualitatively similar to those reported for mixed MPS, indicating a greater potential for protein accretion over time in the UT state. We currently lack information on how MPS increases in the days and weeks (as opposed to hours) after RE and at different times during RT. This type of information would allow a better understanding of how muscle plasticity adapts throughout an RT programme. Specifically, the integrative response of MyoPS should be analysed at temporally distant time points, even days after the performance of heavy RE. Utilization of deuterated water as a tracer could serve this propose [48-50]. Also, to the best of our knowledge, no study to date has tracked MyoPS at multiple times throughout an extended training period; it is worth highlighting that one study did it over a very short period (ie, 8 days [47]), which would seem to be important, as the initial (6 h) MPS response does not correlate with hyper-trophy. Thus, an analysis that captures the behaviour of both variables (ie, MPS integrative data and direct hypertrophic data) over a given training period may better describe the dynamic process of muscle remodeling through RT.[16(806)]*

Note how this paragraph includes impactful conclusive findings and includes the answers to the 2 questions, "What additional research needs to be conducted?" and "Are there questions from this study that need to be addressed?" Some may perceive these questions as limitations (which are discussed below); however, the authors in this subsection only commented on what should happen in the future and not what limited their current study. The conclusions are clearly written in the first 1 or 2 sentences and then the authors guide the reader on what should be done in the future to help augment the progress of medical research on this topic.

Summary

The Conclusion subsection is about creating "bang for the buck" for the reader. For many readers, this subsection is read first to reveal whether the article is relevant to their interest as determined by whether it is a good article, an article worthy of their limited reading time, and if they want to purchase the article.

Limitations Subsection

As another component of the Discussion section, the Limitations subsection allows authors to highlight potential issues with data interpretation as well as why a study cannot be generalized to a larger population. A more refined definition of the Limitations subsection is as follows:

The limitations of the study are those characteristics of design or methodology that impacted or influenced the interpretation of the findings from your research. They are the constraints on generalizability, applications to practice, and/or utility of findings that are the result of the ways in which you initially chose to design the study and/or the method used to establish internal and external validity.[17(p66)]

Manuscript limitations should be focused on those aspects that are inherent to the research problem being investigated. To be clear, every study is limited by time, funding, and resources; however, these are inherent limitations not directly related to the research problem and therefore do not need to be mentioned.

Concerns that can be addressed in a Limitations subsection include sample size/power issues, lack of reliable data, lack of prior research studies on the current topic, self-reported data, access to data, longitudinal effects, and language barriers.[18] In addition, authors may elaborate on different research design concepts that could have been used that would have perhaps allowed for a more complete set of findings, minor design flaws exposed post hoc in the current study, or other unexpected barriers such as a high participant attrition rate. Furthermore, the Limitations subsection should focus on potential biases. For example, in the case of a limitation in subject selection (ie, participant bias), an outcome reported in a particular mouse model may have potentially been influenced by several conditions inherent to that mouse model (eg, obesity, high triglycerides, elevated cholesterol). A limitation could include the lack of a mouse model expressing just the single condition of interest (eg, high triglycerides), therefore suggesting that the condition of interest could be influenced by those other conditions.

Manuscript authors should use the Limitations subsection to outline the study's shortcomings objectively. Thus, limitations should not be viewed as a need to expose weaknesses with the current study but rather manuscript authors should instead emphasize limitations as an opportunity for future research.

Like the Conclusion subsection, structure and style for the Limitations subsection can be somewhat variable. Typically, depending on the author's preference and/or manuscript guidelines, the Limitations subsection appears at the end of the Discussion section. Each limitation should be described in a straight-forward manner with a rationale outlining the reasoning behind the limitation. Once the manuscript author outlines a limitation, he or she should make sure to explain why each limitation could not be overcome in the current study's methodology as well as assess the impact of the limitation on the overall study.[19] However, it is important that researchers address potential limitations during study design in order to reduce the likelihood of their occurrence. Then, if an issue cannot be addressed or was noticed after data collection, it can be addressed as a limitation. For example, patient attrition between pre- and post-treatments cannot always be predicted. If a researcher expects a high attrition rate, it should be addressed during study design by increasing the subject pool. If during the experiment a high attrition rate becomes noticeable and the results are still valid, it may be acceptable to address the high attrition rate in the limitations as a cause for a reduced statistical power or decreased test statistic.

Limitations can be perceived by some as an inherent flaw in a study. Authors must use caution to describe what was lacking or unexplained in their study without appearing as though it was a study design flaw. This in itself can be challenging. First, understand that negative results are not a limitation[20] but may instead indicate that the hypothesis was incorrect. As discussed briefly in Chapter 8, negative results should be presented objectively along with an indication that the hypothesis was incorrect, as even negative data may be useful to some readers. Second, remember to balance results against limitations. Sometimes, a study goes so well that it becomes tempting to generalize the meaning of the results too broadly. Take the time to objectify the limitations regardless if they are positive vs negative and strong vs weak.

Location of the Limitations Subsection

The Limitations subsection can be located in different parts of the Discussion section. Limitations can be written at the beginning, mixed within, or at the end of the Discussion section. Here is an example of an article that addresses limitations at the end of the discussion:

> *Some limitations to this study should be noted. Studies with this many variables (7 sports, 2 sexes, and 12 body parts) are likely to yield "significant" findings based on chance alone. The few statistically significant differences we found between men and women in this study could be explained by this fact. Also, our study did not analyze injury trends over time, a factor which could be valuable when assessing injury patterns. Finally, we were unable to obtain the amount of time lost from sports because of injury, thus losing an opportunity to further assess severity of injury.[21]*

Note that each limitation has its own sentence, is clear and not misleading, and identifies where the limitation may change the outcome of the study. The reader could also appreciate the confounding variables that limit this study but note that the authors kept these limitations simple enough where it does not weaken the overall impact of the article. Yet another example:

> *For instance, a team that competes in the UCL [UEFA Champions League] or EL [European League] tournament, and has no chance of winning the league at a late stage of the season, might put more effort into the final UCL or EL matches and, possibly, less effort into the remaining matches in the league. Consequently, it is a study limitation that domestic cup matches were not included in the analyses, since the results of these matches may also influence a team's performance in the league play and in European cups. UEFA SCC is not solely based on a team's season performance in European cups, as it also includes 20% national association ranking, which is a shortcoming with this measure. Still, it was believed to be a feasible and objective measure of a team's international success, as a complementary measure to the domestic league performance, and the results also followed the same pattern as for domestic performance.[22(p741)]*

In contrast, this group of authors elected to address study limitations throughout their Discussion section. For every result that the authors elaborated on, a subsequent limitation (if present) was adjacent to their statement. This method allows the reader to evaluate a study finding vs its associated limitation. Addressing limitations as done in this example rather than as a distinct subsection contributes to the article's transparency. A final example outlines the placement of the Limitations subsection prior to the Discussion section:

> *The current review was primarily descriptive to provide a comprehensive description with as much of the literature represented as possible. The benefit of such a comprehensive description results in the limitation that a full meta-analytical review could come to stronger conclusions. However, each area of the current review would require a separate meta-analysis and therefore would suffer from not being able to draw on the multifactorial discussion presented in the current review. Furthermore, it should be noted that much of the interpretation of existing studies came from correlational analyses and the readers should consider that correlation does not necessarily indicate causation.[23]*

Being that this is a review article, the authors point out that the narrative review of the literature—rather than another meta-analysis done by the authors—is the limitation. An astute reader would read this as a refresher in knowing that these are inherent limitations in a review article and perceive it as a "known gap." This section serves the purpose of clearing up why one cannot take away from this study more than it presented due to these inherent limitations for the lay reader.

Summary

Remember, the Limitations subsection is a way to show largely unavoidable and/or unexpected issues in a study to allow the reader to make his or her own conclusions about the acceptability of the results. Depending on the limitation(s), they can be written in their own subsection or written throughout the Discussion section. Ultimately manuscript authors should refer to the *Author's Guide* of each journal for instructions.

Clinical Relevance and Practical Applications/Implications

The Clinical Relevance and Practical Applications/Implications subsection is designed to sum up how the findings of a study are going to affect the clinical facet of a particular field such as sports medicine, biomechanics, etc. Oftentimes, Clinical Relevance can serve as an adjunct to the Conclusion. Rather than summarizing the objective findings as might occur in the Conclusion subsection, Clinical Relevance offers a venue to allow for explaining how nonclinical research findings translate into the clinical component of a particular field. The *British Journal of Sports Medicine* offers a unique perspective as it requires a "Summary Box" consisting of 3 to 4 bullet points indicating the new findings outlined in the study results.

The American Journal of Sports Medicine provides guidance for writing the Clinical Relevance section as follows: "[i]f yours was a laboratory study, describe its relevance to clinical sports medicine."[9] These guidelines make it clear that even though a study may have been conducted using basic science techniques, the authors must correlate the relevance of the findings to clinical sports medicine prior to publication in the journal.

Manuscript authors must ensure that they can translate the theoretical/laboratory data into the clinical world by offering a relevance statement. For example, there are multiple animal studies showing that nonsteroidal anti-inflammatory drugs (NSAIDs) may slow down bone healing in stress fractures, along with studies that contradict this statement. These original studies conducted using basic science techniques could, at the time of publication, extrapolate the "clinical relevance" of using Tylenol over NSAIDs in stress-fractured human patients.[24] Further studies confirming this association in humans should of course be mentioned in the Conclusion subsection as a potential recommendation for future research.

Closely related to the Clinical Relevance subsection is the Practical Application or Implications subsection, which blends in Limitations, Clinical Relevance, and Conclusion in a unique matter. The goal of this section depends on the journal type. For example, in the *International Journal of Sports Physiology and Performance*,

> The Practical Applications section is an important feature of manuscripts published in *International Journal of Sports Physiology and Performance*. Authors should summarize how the findings could be useful for coaches and athletes and/or other researchers in sport physiology and sport performance. The study's limitations and generalizability should also be addressed and, where necessary, recommendations made for future research.[25(p3)]

In another example, the *Journal of Science and Medicine in Sport* states,

> Practical Implications—3 to 5 dot (bulleted) points summarizing the practical findings derived from the study to the real-world setting of sport and exercise—that can be understood by a lay audience. Avoid overly scientific terms and abbreviations. Dot points should not include recommendations for further research.[26(p9)]

These 2 journals (*Journal of Science and Medicine in Sport* and *International Journal of Sports Physiology and Performance*) recommend that Practical Implications be written as an individual subsection. The former editor-in-chief of the *Journal of Science and Medicine in Sport*, Gregory S. Kolt, elaborates on this section indirectly:

> In many respects, research findings are only as valuable as how well they can be put into practice to improve outcomes. Whether the outcome is the elimination of a disease, the prevention of an injury, rehabilitation and return to sport and physical activity, or improving the efficiency and performance of sport and exercise skills, we often require guidance from the vast literature as to how to put rather complex findings into practice. With a rapidly increasing volume of published literature in many areas of sports medicine and sports science, some sense needs to be made of it through guiding statements and summaries that assist in the application to benefit those we work with. It is important, however, that such summaries are based on the best available evidence and are presented with a balanced perspective.[27(p251)]

In the world of sports medicine as well as kinesiology, the Practical Applications subsection is useful for a specific type reader who is interested in how or whether a particular finding has relevance in the clinical setting. For example, a recent article was published on self-reported balance status in adolescents at 1-month post-concussion.

> When taking care of adolescents in the training room post-concussion that are a few weeks from their injury, the injured athlete may have balance defects regardless of if they believe or not. Balance examination regardless of the athlete's belief on his balance will offer better insight into their deficits.[28]

In the above statement, there is a blend of the Conclusion as well as the Clinical Relevance subsections; however, if read by a coach, athletic trainer, or athlete, this statement remains easy to understand. Of note, the example given[22] in the Clinical Relevance section about European soccer injuries may also fit this definition. The similarity in these 2 examples is that the content is addressing a similar audience. In contrast, the Practical Applications subsection gives a narrower statement that reflects the study whereas the Clinical Relevance subsection is more translational and generalized.

Summary

The writing style of the Clinical Relevance and Practical Applications/Implications subsections should match the style of the rest of the manuscript, be original in statement (as this is the only section in which you can "translate" laboratory medicine into the clinical world), and keep it short without embellishment.

Conclusion

As described, the subsections outlined in this chapter serve to allow the manuscript author more freedom to elaborate their narrative within a study or a particular section of the IMRaD format to provide a concise description for the reader. There is overlap in how these subsections are formatted within the IMRaD sections and between each other as shown above. Specific to the contrasting writing styles, content, and giving examples of how to format each section, this chapter will hopefully serve as a guide to enhance the writing capabilities of manuscript authors.

References

1. Glasman-Deal H. *Science Research Writing: A Guide for Non-Native Speakers of English*. London, England: Imperial College Press; 2009.
2. Hall G. *How to Write a Paper*. 5th ed. Oxford, England: BMJ Books; 2012.
3. Singer AJ, Hollander JE. How to write a manuscript. *J Emerg Med*. 2009;36:89-93.
4. Calver N. Sir Peter Medawar: science, creativity and the popularization of Karl Poper. *Notes and Records of the Royal Society of London*. 2013;67(4):301-314.
5. Howitt S, Wilson A. Revisiting "Is the scientific paper a fraud?". *EMBO Reports*. 2014;15(5):481-484.
6. International Committee of Medical Journal Editors. Uniform requirements of manuscripts submitted to biomedical journals. http://www.icmje.org/urm_full.pdf. Published April 2010.
7. Kotur PF. How to write a scientific article for a medical journal. *Indian J Anaesth*. 2002;46(1):21-25.
8. Borja A. 11 steps to structuring a science paper editors will take seriously. https://www.elsevier.com/connect/11-steps-to-structuring-a-science-paper-editors-will-take-seriously. Published June 24, 2014. Accessed June 21, 2018.
9. AJSM manuscript submission guidelines. American Journal of Sports Medicine. http://journals.sagepub.com/pb-assets/cmscontent/AJS/AJSM_Submission_Guidelines.pdf.
10. A concise format for reporting the longer-term follow-up status of patients managed with arthroplasty at any joint. *Journal of Bone & Joint Surgery*. http://journals.lww.com/jbjsjournal/Pages/Concise-Format-Guidelines.aspx.
11. Belcher W. *Writing Your Journal Article in 12 Weeks: A Guide to Academic Publishing*. Thousand Oaks, CA: Sage; 2009.
12. Feak CB, Swales JM. *Academic Writing for Graduate Students*. Ann Arbor, MI: University of Michigan Press; 1994.
13. Partridge B, Starfield S. *Thesis and Dissertation Writing in a Second Language: A Handbook for Supervisors*. Abingdon, England: Routledge; 2007.
14. Kumar K, Mandleywala S, Gannon M, Estes N, Weinstock J, Link M. Development of a chest wall protector effective in preventing sudden cardiac death by chest wall impact (commotio cordis). *Clin J Sports Med*. 2007;27(1):26-30.
15. Longo U, Ciuffreda M, Loche J, Berton A, Salvatore G, Denaro V. Treatment of primary acute patellar dislocation: systematic review and quantitative synthesis of the literature. *Clin J Sports Med*. 2017;27(6):511-523.
16. Damas F, Phillips S, Vechin FC, Ugrinowitsch C. A review of resistance training-induced changes in skeletal muscle protein synthesis and their contribution to hypertrophy. *Sports Medicine*. 2015;45:801-807.
17. Pierce JH, Murnan J. Research limitations and the necessity of reporting them. *Am J Health Educ*. 2004;35:66-67.
18. Brutus S, Aguinis H, Wassmer U. Self-reported limitations and future directions in scholarly reports analysis and recommendations. *Journal of Management*. 2013;39(1):48-75.
19. Aguinis H, Edwards JR. Methodical wishes for the next decade and how to make wishes come true. *J Manag Stud*. 2014;51(1):143-174.
20. Lewis GH, Lewis JF. The dog in the night-time: negative evidence in social research. *Br J Sociol*. 1980;31:544-558.
21. Sallis, RE, Jones K, Sunshine S, Smith G, Simon, G. Comparing sports injuries in men and women. *Int J Sports Med*. 2001;22:420-423.
22. Hagglund M, Walden M, Magnusson H, Kristenson K, Bengtsson H, Ekstrand J. Injuries affect team performance negatively in professional football: an 11-year follow-up of the UEFA Champions League injury study. *Br J Sports Med*. 2013;47:738-742.
23. Suchomel TJ, Nimphius S, Stone MH. The importance of muscular strength in athletic performance. *Sports Med*. 2016;46:1419-1449.
24. Pountos I, Georgouli T, Giannoudis PV. Do nonsteroidal anti-inflammatory drugs affect bone healing? A critical analysis. *The Scientific World Journal*. doi:10.1100/2012/606404.
25. Author guidelines. *International Journal of Sports Physiology and Performance*. http://journals.humankinetics.com/page/authors/ijspp. Accessed June 21, 2018.
26. Author info. *Journal of Science and Medicine in Sport*. http://www.jsams.org/content/authorinfo. Accessed June 21, 2018.
27. Kolt G. Practical applications of research findings. *J Sci Med Sport*. 2009;12(2):251.
28. Rochefort C, Walters-Stewart C, Aglipay M, Barrowman N, Zemek R, Sveistrup H. Self-reported balance status is not a reliable indicator of balance performance in adolescents at one-month post-concussion. *J Sci Med Sport*. 2017;20(11):970-975.

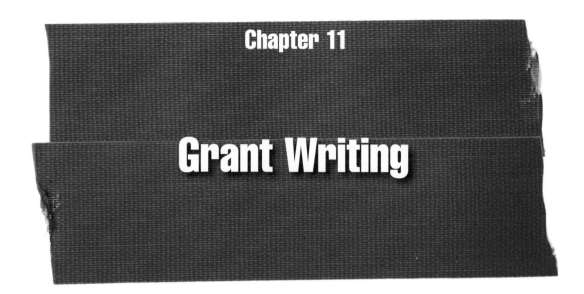

Thomas Lowder, PhD

Introduction

I'm Supposed to Pay for This Myself?

Well, the short answer to any researcher asking that question is *yes*. Grant-writing expectations for faculty members run the gamut from the requirement that researchers will apply for internal grants at the college-level (meaning that the researcher's own institution has a few thousand dollars available to perform a small project) to earning one's summer salary through an external grant. At some institutions—particularly major research or medical institutions—it may be that a grant pays for half of the researcher's salary; all of his or her summer salary; and a lab full of students, post-doctoral fellows, and a lab tech to keep everything running smoothly while the principal investigator (PI) is seeking even more funding by writing more grants. At many of these institutions, a researcher's grant-writing ability can mean the difference between having a summer income and managing to survive on half-pay, since many institutions pay researchers on a 9-month contract, meaning no paychecks are received in the summer outside of those paid for through a research grant.

Will My Grant Be Funded?

"Is it fundable?" is an oft-asked question in scientific discussions. This is often more of a deciding factor as to whether the work is something that a researcher might be passionate about or even care about. There are more than a few successful researchers who study and publish cutting-edge research that they do not particularly feel strongly about, but the fact remains that cutting-edge research is what pays the bills. The rationale behind this mentality is "to pay for my lab, do the work that I'm being paid to do, and then I will be able to do all of the projects I really want to do on the side" (Sidebars 11-1 and 11-2).

Knoblauch M. *Professional Writing in Kinesiology and Sports Medicine* (pp 111-126).
© 2019 Taylor & Francis Group.

Sidebar 11-1

Not every grant stipulates that the researcher has to perform the exact work he or she is proposing. Rather, the overriding requirement is that the money is spent in pursuit of science.

Sidebar 11-2

A logical follow-up question to "Is it fundable?" that any researcher should ask is, "Do I *want* to do this work?" Many researchers experience a change in their career trajectory because they are able to do research for which they can receive funding. This does not necessarily mean that this is the work they want to do, but rather the work they have to do. A very good friend of mine funds his lab because he received funding from a very generous federal agency for some simple but basic (for him) experiments. Since he was successful with his first grant, he has been fortunate to have maintained this line of funding for some time. He is, however, moderately unenthused with this work as his passions lay elsewhere. Nonetheless, he is able to pay for his lab and hire post-doctoral fellows and graduate students, and he can still do some of his more exciting work on the side.

All researchers will have to find a starting point for their grant. For example, many new researchers will continue or segue from some of their recent (eg, post-doctoral, PhD, etc) experiments. Doing so will allow them to remain in their comfort zone where they have likely had at least some success (publications, small or even National Institute of Health [NIH] pre-/post-doctoral grants). Furthermore, continuing along a particular research line increases the likelihood that they know how to do "the next step" as they have likely described those very next steps in prior publications (eg, the Future Directions section of previous manuscripts). In almost every case, the researcher applying for a grant will have to convince the funding agency that he or she can do the work outlined in the grant proposal and that he or she has the network and resources (discussed later) to support the work. Therefore, the logical step for many researchers is to stay within their comfort zone and write grants that they feel quite comfortable with in terms of understanding the methods and completing the project.

Alternatively, researchers may choose to step out of their comfort zone. Doing so can be a gamble. A researcher may have a wealth of preliminary data to show that the experiment "should" work, but this pathway can be risky. Why? If a PI works on a project that is familiar to him or her, he or she has the "safety" of knowing what he or she is doing. However, the PI may also run the risk of effectively repeating previous experiments when he or she was a PhD student or post-doctoral fellow. This may be a safe bet toward a favorable outcome, but will the researcher impress the reviewers with cutting-edge science? Unless the researcher proposes the "next logical step" in his or her previous work, probably not. The stepping-out part involves balancing risk and reward—proposing work that may not have been done before, but may have a high reward, such as a new technique to better analyze tumor progression. The problem, of course, is that now the researcher has entered into the confounding "I have never done this before, and have to convince the powers-that-be that I know what I am doing" area of research. This is where his or her skills as a convincing storyteller will be highlighted in the grant writing process. This is also where the researcher finds out if he or she is able to find collaborators who may help with the research, or at the very least serve as a mentor on the grant.

Perhaps a researcher is proposing a series of experiments that will require a new technique that has not been tried before, or use a new experimental model that has not been looked at yet.

Sidebar 11-3

David "Deacon" Jones was a very successful pass rusher in the NFL and is considered to be one of the architects for creating the "quarterback sack" before there was such a term. When he would teach younger players how to play his position, he stated that playing defensive line was like water: take the path of least resistance. If only science were so easy. The problem, of course, is that we do not always want our research path dictated to us. When planning out your grant, try taking the path of most resistance—what obstacles must you overcome to get to where you want to be? Like Sisyphus pushing that huge boulder up the hill only to have it roll down again every day, you will have more than a few hardships and obstacles to overcome. The more you push that boulder up the hill, the more obstacles you will remove for your grant reviewers.

This is where the researcher's passion must come in to the writing. If the researcher is proposing a rather risky set of experiments with a likely—but not guaranteed—outcome, that researcher's writing must impart a reassurance that yes, the research design **will** work, in words that 2 or 3 grant reviewers will understand. Convincing reviewers of a risky set of experiments is rather bold, particularly for a young scientist (more on this later). In contrast, this is also something that is valued for its novelty and cutting-edge appeal (Sidebar 11-3).

The Process of Review

The grant review process is more or less the same with all grants, be they federal, foundation, or society grants, and even small institutional grants. Similar to a playground game where kids pick teams, grant applications are going to be ranked and reviewed in front of other scientists, some of whom may be people the researcher knows directly. Often, these grant reviews are conducted by people who know little about the particular work that a researcher conducts. This in turn high-lights the importance of a researcher's writing to effectively communicate the premise of his or her grant. While the process is supposed to be institutionalized (meaning that there is a more-or-less standard way of assessing and scoring grants) and efficient, to an applicant, it can feel anything but organized. "That reviewer didn't understand what I was trying to say" or "I discussed this in the introduction!" are among the many frustrations researchers experience after finding out that they were not funded, and they often blame the reviewers for not catching it because it is the reviewer's fault, right? Well, not so much. Researchers should never assume that their work will be understood. Just like any person can see last night's dream in his or her head, if he or she tries to explain that dream to someone and that person does not picture it the way intended, getting mad at that person will not help. Rather, time must be spent in order to draw a clearer picture—time which may not exist.

It is the grant applicant's job to outline for those reviewers a project that they can follow, written by an expert (ie, the researcher) and read by someone who understands but may or may not be an expert in the researcher's field (ie, the grant review team). If a researcher cannot clearly explain to the reviewers what he or she proposes to do, that is an error in the researcher's writing and not an error in the reviewer's understanding. The reviewers want to advocate for grant applicants; money is available, and it will be disbursed to someone. The key of course is for the PI to convince the review team that the PI should be one of those who should be funded. Unfortunately, the only avenue that the PI has to convince the review team is through his or her grant application because, as mentioned, grant reviewers want to advocate for a qualified researcher. Therefore, if an application is written in a way that the reviewers can sell, they will try their best to sell it to the grant review team on which they sit.

Sidebar 11-4

When I was a post-doctoral fellow, my advisor offered a course simply entitled "Grant Writing"; obviously an important course. Of the 30 or so post-doctoral fellows enrolled in this course, about two-thirds of us were submitting a grant (mostly F31 NIH fellowships). Those of us who were actively writing prior to the course being offered were fortunate (gulp) enough to have our grants reviewed by NIH study section members—in front of everyone. I had heard how grants were reviewed—multiple reviewers sitting around a giant table with stacks of grants while 2 or 3 reviewers summarized all of those months of writing in just a couple of minutes. Scientifically, I had never felt so naked in my life. ALL of the work that I put into writing that was shared, the good and bad, by 2 reviewers who matter-of-factly read what I was planning on doing, the odds of it working, and the mistakes I made. Each reviewer spent 3 to 4 minutes doing this and it was on to the next one. To say it was an eye-opener as to how analytical and processed this method was is an understatement to say the least. This is the process, and I realized that those 2 or 3 people are the only ones I needed to convince. Fortunately, I received funding; that is a high that we all chase.

Preparing the Grant

Getting All the Help Possible

Having run the gamut from "successful" grant writer to "well, not so much," there are a few words of wisdom that this chapter's author can impart that become particularly relevant here. The first is that "successful" is quite liberally defined in many circles. By definition, a successful grant is one that is funded. However, not having a grant funded does not necessarily mean failure; oftentimes, grants are submitted and then reworked, sometimes exhaustively, for resubmission. This of course means that it may be an additional grant cycle (about 4 months) or 2 until the grant is resubmitted. Having someone knowledgeable in grantsmanship—either someone who has had several funded grants or, better still, someone sitting on a grant review (ie, "study section")—read the prepared grant can help markedly (Sidebar 11-4).

Making a Plan

Everyone wants to conduct original and cutting-edge research. Anyone who does not is not really conducting research but rather is repeating prior experiments. How a researcher chooses his or her research is up to him or her, but before one can set out for a destination, he or she must know where to go. Simply packing a bag, getting in a car, and driving might sound like a good idea, but there are lot of red flags with this approach. Questions that need to be asked of a researcher prior to beginning the writing of their grant include:

- How do you know where you are going? Without a point on the map, you might find yourself lost, perhaps in an unfriendly environment. This of course relates to writing specific aims. A bit of discussion about the Aims page is found later in this chapter as the Specific Aims page is the key to a successful grant, or so many researchers have been told.
- Did you pack appropriately? If you packed for the beach and you are headed to North Dakota in January, you might find yourself ill-equipped for such a hostile environment. This means the right funding agency; is your grant appropriate for these folks?
- Is your car well-maintained? Running out of resources is never a good idea. Lab/university resources include equipment, personnel, a "go-to" person as either a collaborator and/or mentor, or institutional support.

- Is your car designed for the journey? You may write the grant, but if you were to get it, are **you** prepared for the grant? Do you have the training, resources, time, and expertise to perform this work?

How Do I Start Writing My Grant?

This is the million-dollar question, or the "$275,000 plus indirect costs" question, if aiming for a smaller R21 grant. To answer simply, any researcher who has generated data has already started writing his or her grant. This initial effort can be used as preliminary data to look at a "bigger picture" project, which usually requires a proposal for funding in the way of a grant. Hopefully the research proposed is also at least slightly different from all other applicants, which will help to make that researcher's work stand out (Sidebar 11-5).

Most grant applicants probably started their grant by reading a paper or looking at an experiment being conducted while wondering, "Why didn't I measure that?" or by chatting with a colleague. This is the fun part of science, the "no one has done this before." Unfortunately, it can also serve to make one's job as a researcher a bit more difficult. The old saying of "research is what we do when we do not know what we are doing" is applicable. Researchers want to perform a set of experiments that are similar to other work in the literature but have not yet been published or presented previously. This means the researcher has to demonstrate proficiency in what has been done (ie, a literature review) as well as what has not been done specific to conducting their experiment (ie, developing a quality Methods section). More simply put, a researcher's writing needs to convince a grant review team that, while he or she has not done this work (nor has anyone else), the researcher has the requisite skills and support needed to accomplish what is written in the grant proposal, within the allotted time and budget, using a technique that may not have been developed or published yet.

Outlining the Idea

When writing a research manuscript, the research has already been conducted and the researcher knows the end results. The premise of a research grants is different because no results are known and the researcher must therefore outline clearly and concisely what he or she *expects* to happen. As the idea for a grant begins to take shape, a researcher will outline his or her idea(s) internally (ie, with him- or herself) at first. No one wants to sound like an idiot, particularly in front of colleagues, so most likely the initial work is reworked and reformatted repeatedly. It is important that researchers try to punch as many holes in their own arguments as possible; if they do not, the grant review team certainly will (and excess "holes" will result in no chance at funding). After outlining the main premise or concepts of the grant, the researcher's next discussion will likely be with a colleague who knows the researcher's work and is familiar with what they do, such as a graduate student, mentor, etc (Sidebar 11-6).

Structuring the Writing to the Funding Agency

Each funding agency is different in why they are soliciting grants, and grant writers must ensure that the premise of their grant is aligned with the intent of the funding agency. The NIH is concerned with good science; they want to fund the best science (ie, the "best" grants) that they review. Private funding agencies, such as foundations, may have a different goal. Foundations are often small organizations with few resources, including money. They may read a grant that is very technology-driven and contains great science, but this may not be in line with the goal of their agency. Often, the small foundations are looking for immediate impact and something they can show as "we funded a study that found xxx treatment benefits our patients, and here is why … "

What (and How) to Write—AKA, Your Checklist

While the concept of writing a grant is relatively simple, the process is actually quite detailed. For large (eg, R01) grants, it is not uncommon to turn in a 100-or-more–page proposal (12 pages of the actual grant) with near log-scale that amount in supplementary paperwork such as additional personnel, budgets, letters of support, and pictures of you in front of your lab holding a sign reading "Will pipet for (grant) money" that takes weeks or months to generate. Even smaller foundation-based grants require extensive detail that will necessitate collaboration with other researchers as well as the institutional grant office. For example, most grants will require information specific to:

- Breakdown of the sections, subsections, and other parts of the grant
- Biographies of everyone involved with the grant
- Equipment list(s) and available resources, including personnel and "go to" people for help
- Curriculum vitae (formatted to the agencies you are submitting your grants to)
- Stylistic points (eg, writing tone, varying formats, visuals, font, etc)

That last bullet point—writing style—is important. Does it make sense to all relevant parties and is it written in a proper tone? That is, will the reviewer(s) understand the writing? If a researcher's colleagues who understand the science and a colleague who is not familiar with the science come to roughly the same conclusion about what will be done, the researcher has successfully written for a wide audience. Keep this in mind: a researcher staring at the same grant for months will understand it quite differently than someone given a copy of the grant who is unfamiliar with it.

The bulk of a researcher's writing time will likely be spent on the first bullet point above: writing the individual sections of the grant. Most federal grants (eg, R01, R21, etc) follow a specific format, while smaller foundational grants typically have individual formats for each grant. However, researchers will ultimately find consistency between grants for specific sections, many of which are outlined next.

Literature Review

A researcher writing a grant knows the literature probably as well, if not better, than anyone. A PI just starting his or her career will be the best-read person as a result of his or her dissertation committee or post-doctoral advisor having had the PA read "everything." By knowing the literature, the researcher can answer the question, "Has this been done before?" to which the answer will be, "Of course not, or else there would not be a reason for doing these experiments." There are similar designs out there that can provide much of a researcher's rationale.

Reviewers read, too. This is why they are a part of the review team. Of course many of the reviewers who will read the PI's grant *are the literature*, meaning that they have published and have been successful in receiving grants and are therefore well-versed in what comprises a fundable grant vs one that is scored but not funded (or not even reviewed). Because the review team is well versed in the literature, it is important that the researcher's proposal exhibit brevity. Researchers do not have much space in a grant and as such do not want nor need to retell their dissertation literature review. They may only have a few paragraphs (with a lot of references) to explain an entire body of prior work. Learning to write concisely while thoroughly explaining everything is truly an art form, and the only way to be a good artist is to practice one's craft.

Specific Aims and Sub-Aims

The Specific Aims page is the grant's starting and ending point as it outlines precisely what the researcher intends to do. Specific aims could probably be called *exact aims* as they must lay out in exquisite detail what will be done in order to achieve a certain outcome through manipulation or intervention of a specific population, target, cell, etc, and quantifiably assess what impact the treatment had on a very specific variable. A well-written Specific Aims page must summarize what has and has not been done in the field, convince the reviewer that the grant will address at least one important area that has not been addressed in the field, and also convince the reviewer that the work will be done in such a way that it will be replicable and reproducible. The exact set of experiments (to be discussed in concise and precise detail in the later grant pages) will be summarized in the specific aims (with **bolded** and occasionally *italicized* keywords for effect).

Because of its importance, the Specific Aims page is the page that researchers will spend probably 40% of their time writing and editing. Without a perfect (or near-perfect) Aims page from which everything flows, a researcher will not be funded (Sidebar 11-7).

There may be 2 or 3 (or more) specific aims in a researcher's proposal, depending on the size and scope of the grant. A general rule is to generate 2 specific aims that are related but NOT dependent upon each other. That is, Aim 1 is relative to Aim 2 in that they support one another, but Aim 2 does not rely on the successful completion of Aim 1. If the aims are dependent upon each other, reviewers will most likely question the grant because the grant's success becomes dependent upon both aims of the grant working properly. "All or nothing" is not always wise in grantsmanship. Providing separate but related aims provides a "safety net" so that if one aim (ie, the primary aim) does not pan out, the other is still fully operational.

The Specific Aims page will have a concise but very well-thought out line or 2 that outlines the major purpose of the part(s) of the grant that will be investigated. The sub-aims are those little

Sidebar 11-7

Down the hall from my lab was our resident grant guru. This individual had continual R01 (ie, federal grant) funding for decades and, on more than a few occasions, scored grants in the single percentiles, meaning one of the best grants reviewed for that particular study section. During a brief hallway chat, he inquired about my grant progress. I was a little embarrassed to tell him that I was stuck on my specific aims. I knew what I wanted to say, I explained, but I felt lost since I could not get this into a few sentences. He knowingly grinned and told me that meant I was doing well. Now thoroughly confused, I asked what he meant. "I spend roughly half of my time on the specific aims page, most of it on those 2 or 3 very specific aims," he told me. In discussing this with my advisor, she reaffirmed this. Every reviewer will use the specific aims page as their base of support. This is the one page that is thumb-marked while reading the entire grant, and that nondominant thumb is probably, for easy reference, touching that first specific aim. Make it very easy for the reviewer and do not deviate from these aims. This is THE starting and finishing point, and the one page that the reviewers will keep their thumb on while reading the grant. Whatever aim(s) proposed, these had better match, exactly, anything stated within the grant. All of the writing within the grant must flow back to these specific aims. Writing a successful grant is similar to firing an arrow at a target: the further away the target is, the more that can go wrong. Grants are like targets; even if the aims and everything else is lined up dead-center, there are a lot of things that can cause the arrow to miss the target. There is no such thing as a "small" grant anymore, meaning those smaller (ie, non-NIH grants) have become very competitive as well. Everyone puts their best (hopefully) efforts into every grant. Reviewers need to find a reason to rank someone's grant higher or lower than another PI's grant. Deviating from the specific aims may be just the thing to do if the PI intends to sink his or her chances of funding.

parts below these bolded aims sections that include the 2, 4, or even more sets of experiments that will be performed independently to form an answer for the primary aims. These sub-aims may include secondary goals of the grant that are important but not the number one priority of the research grant. An example might be that if Aim 1 proposes to use a new technique to analyze cell proliferation in real time, "a secondary aim of Aim 1 will be to determine if analysis of this same tumor line will yield identical results in the mediastinal lymph node as seen in the primary target organ—the lung—and if these results correlate with less-invasive measures, such as venous blood."

Sample Specific Aims Page

Following is a sample Aims page from a successful (ie, funded) NIH F32 post-doctoral grant looking at cellular response to exercise in an asthma model. Each grant is constructed differently; therefore, authors must ensure that their application is relevant to the particular framework of the particular grant. Understand also that what is written here is the "final product"; half of what was originally proposed was ultimately changed or eliminated from the aims (Sidebar 11-8).

I. Specific Aims: The overarching hypothesis of this proposal is that moderate-intensity aerobic exercise training attenuates asthma pathogenesis through increased regulatory T (T_{reg}) cell responses *in vivo*. The aims to test this hypothesis include:

A. Specific Aim #1: Determine the effects of moderate-intensity aerobic exercise training on T_{reg} cell phenotype in a murine model of asthma. Hypothesis. Moderate-intensity aerobic exercise training increases the population of CD4+CD25+Foxp3+ T_{reg} cells within a murine asthma model. Experimental Approach. Foxp3^{EGFP} reporter mice will be sensitized with either ovalbumin (OVA) or control saline and exercised at a moderate intensity using a motorized treadmill; sedentary control mice will be permitted free movement within their cages.

Sidebar 11-8

I would love to say that the reason my grant was funded on the first submission was due to its outstanding Specific Aims page (along with its brilliance and cutting-edge technology). While I do think that it was well-written, a large part of the success of that grant was also due to timing. *Timing* here means that a fair amount of what is current, or trending, can often have a major effect on what is prioritized. If a grant is submitted that proposes to reduce transmission of Ebola virus by using a new saliva test kit and there happens to be a series of Ebola outbreaks in Africa, this may benefit your grant. However, if your grant proposes to assess the function of that same test when an established (and more accurate) test has just come to market, your grant may be negatively affected. The lab that I was working in when I submitted the grant had an established record of using exercise to reduce airway hyper-responsiveness and lung inflammation in a mouse model of asthma, and working at a major medical research center did not hurt. Also, critically, regulatory T cells were undergoing a resurgence in the scientific literature at the time.

Upon completion of the OVA-sensitization and exercise training regimen, CD4$^+$ T cells will be isolated from spleen and lung tissues and examined for changes in Foxp3 reporter (EGFP) expression and T_{reg} cell-related surface markers, including CD25, CD152, and membrane-bound TGF-beta.

B. Specific Aim #2: Determine the effects of moderate-intensity aerobic exercise training on T_{reg} cell function in a murine model of asthma. <u>Hypothesis</u>. Moderate-intensity aerobic exercise training attenuates asthma-related responses by enhancing T_{reg} cell function. <u>Experimental Approach</u>. Foxp3^{EGFP} reporter mice will be sensitized with either OVA or saline and exercised on a motorized treadmill at a moderate intensity; control mice will be permitted free movement within their cages. Upon conclusion of the OVA-sensitization and exercise training protocol, CD4$^+$CD25$^+$Foxp3$^+$ T_{reg} cells will be isolated from spleen and lung tissues and examined for differences in proliferation. In addition, studies will determine their effectiveness in suppressing: i) T cell proliferation *in vitro*; and ii) Th2 responses, airway eosinophilia, and airway hyper-responsiveness (AHR) *in vivo*.

C. Rationale:

Why determine the effects of moderate intensity aerobic training on T_{reg} cell responses? Aerobic exercise training profoundly affects the immune system, including T cell responses.[1] Specifically, aerobic exercise training promotes the redistribution of T lymphocytes between the periphery and vasculature and decreases the ratios of CD4:CD8 as well as naïve:memory T cells *in vivo*.[2] The effects of aerobic exercise training on the responses of T_{reg} cells, however, have not been elucidated. *We present preliminary data in this proposal that suggest moderate-intensity aerobic exercise training increases T_{reg} cell responses in OVA-sensitized mice.*

Why determine the effects of moderate-intensity aerobic exercise training on T_{reg} cell responses in asthma? Asthma has increased in prevalence, morbidity and mortality over the past 20 years.[3] Several clinical studies have reported that aerobic exercise training improves cardiovascular fitness and the general quality of life for asthmatics[1,4,5]; however, the effects of aerobic exercise training on specific T_{reg} cell-related responses are not fully appreciated. Increasing evidence demonstrates that T lymphocytes, including CD4$^+$CD25$^+$Foxp3$^+$ naturally occurring T_{reg} (N-T_{reg}) cells, play a central role in suppressing asthma pathogenesis. Specifically, the CD4$^+$CD25$^+$Foxp3$^+$ N-T_{reg} cell population has previously been shown to inhibit Th2 responses, airway eosinophilia, and allergen-induced AHR.[6,7] We have previously reported that, in OVA-sensitized mice, moderate-intensity aerobic exercise training attenuates lung inflammation and airway remodeling via a mechanism that involves endogenous

> ## Sidebar 11-9
>
> Now it is time for teachable moments and words of wisdom regarding specific aims. One, your specific aims are not your life's work. This is a grant proposal. This will change—the contents, the methodology, perhaps even (dare I say) the aims. You may have written your grant around a set of specific aims only to realize later that those aims are terrible and need to be rewritten. Do not feel as if you have failed at this point. More than likely, you have succeeded in that you have figured a better way to state what you want to measure. Keep that big idea in mind: you may have changed your aims from attempting to block histamine production in an asthma model to attempting to reduce mast cell degranulation in that same model. Your end result is still the same for the patient, that of decreased airway inflammation and hypersensitivity. Do not be so attached to your specific aims that you are not willing to rewrite or even replace them when needed.

glucocorticoids.[8,9] *In this proposal, we present preliminary data that demonstrate that moderate-intensity aerobic exercise training suppresses Th2 responses, airway eosinophilia, and AHR in OVA-sensitized mice.*

It is anticipated that the proposed experiments will permit a thorough examination of the effects of moderate-intensity aerobic exercise training on T_{reg} cell phenotype and function as well as the role of T_{reg} cells in exercise-mediated attenuation of asthma-related responses in vivo.

Written under the constraints of a grant proposal, this Aims page would indeed be 1 page (if using the maximum allowable margins of 0.5"). This is not a coincidence. The Aims page is the "everything" page. This is everyone's starting point, jump-off point, and reset page for reviewers. What is the grant about? See Aims page. How will these experiments be conducted? See Aims page. No work that has already been performed will be stated in this section. In addition, any future work that will be performed will be listed here. (Note that this does not mean the entire methodology, which may take pages, will be listed in the aims. The small moving parts will not be covered in the aims, just the fact that the car is going down the road in a specific direction.) The importance of the Aims page cannot be stated strongly enough, and this comes from someone who despises using "cannot be stated strongly enough." If this page is a mess, do not submit (Sidebar 11-9).

Preliminary Data

Many, perhaps most, grants do not require preliminary data, but it is rare that grants will be funded without at least a bit of evidence demonstrating that the researcher can actually do the work and show encouraging data regarding the experiment he or she is proposing to do. Within the grant application, it is imperative that the applicant show enough evidence that the work will most likely be successful, yet he or she also does not want to do the experiment before submitting the grant. (This does happen frequently.) Show the data and tell a story using both the writing and the graphs, figures, and tables, and focus on writing in a way that will explain how the work will move the field forward (Sidebar 11-10).

Space is limited in a grant. As is the case with the literature review section, it is important that the researcher not retell an entire field with figures and graphs. For example, if trying to receive funding by proposing a new method for reducing influenza viral replication *in vivo*, the grant applicant does not need to discuss the policies of childhood vaccination in reducing the economic cost of lost job productivity due to parents missing work while caring for their child. A few quality stand-alone graphs or figures can often provide enough data to justify a large portion of the grant. Keep these components simple and well thought out. If the preliminary data are confusing, odds are the reviewers will also be confused, and that can be fatal for a grant application.

"Preliminary data may be included but are not required." Uh huh. Preliminary data are one way in which that dream of grant receipt can be explained, rather easily, in picture (or table/graph/plot) form. Outlining preliminary data can be one of the absolute best ways to convince reviewers that you can, in fact, perform these risky and bold experiments. If you have a figure, or 3, that demonstrate competency in a technique or assay that is not in your previous body of work, this will help to alleviate concerns. It is your job to propose a novel but feasible set of experiments that can be completed in the time frame you have put forth and with the resources you have available and the monies that will be awarded to you. This is not always easier said than done. You may be able to perform this work; preliminary data—or better still, a publication or one in press—will affirm that you are indeed capable of doing this type of science. Perhaps you have an antibody that no one else has access to, and this will allow your grant to stand out. If you do not have this antibody but know of someone who does, more than likely your grant will be a collaborative effort involving coinvestigators on your grant. Ultimately, you will have to convince these reviewers that you can do the work you are proposing.

Materials and Methods

What is going to be done and *how* is the researcher going to do it? This is the section from which a study will be "sold" to the review team. How the work will be performed (along with collecting and analyzing data) should all be written in a way that will convince 2 or 3 reviewers that the grant should be put at the top of the other dozen or hundred grants, particularly if this is an innovative method or a complex analysis that is not commonly used. Therefore, researchers should write this section to the audience. In the case of most large grants, the audience will likely be a group of scientists in lay-science, meaning these are readers who know the work but perhaps not the particulars. The tone of the grant should ensure that the reviewers can be educated without becoming bored. Researchers will have an idea of who might read their grant if they are able to submit their grant to the study section requested, but it is not a guarantee that a grant will be sent to a particular section. Most likely, established researchers who know science, and perhaps the field, will be on the grant review section.

Timeline

As if they were not busy enough already, researchers must also be adept at scheduling. With any grant application, one can expect to need to develop a detailed timeline that outlines the course of events in which particular milestones of the proposed experiment will be reached. Furthermore, reviewers will evaluate and critique the proposed timeline. Is the outlined set of experiments feasible in the time allotted? If one proposes to assess the life cycle of drosophila, 1 year is adequate. If the aim is to examine the aging process of a tortoise, perhaps the researcher should not aim for a 1-year time frame.

Specific to the timeline, a number of variables should be factored in. If a PI is at an R1 institution, research is the tail that wags the dog, of course. More than likely, the researcher's department chair will bend over backwards to find resources such as a reduced teaching load if awarded an R01. What if the researcher is at a smaller institution with a moderate or even heavy teaching/service load that will require much more of his or her time? Many times, funding agencies demand a protected (guaranteed) amount of time for the researcher to carry out the work outlined in the awarded grant. A researcher may ultimately need a letter from the chair (or dean) with written support of protected time for this grant.

Budget

Odds are that most researchers did not have a whole lot of business courses during their doctoral or post-doctoral years. This can be unfortunate because budgets can be terrible beasts. Before a researcher realizes it, all of the money that was meant trying to conduct the science has been utilized for salaries, equipment, personnel, and other costs, with no money left over for science. For example, just the salary area of a budget must account for the following:

- Graduate and/or undergraduate student salaries plus fringe (check into work study for undergraduate students as this may save some funds)
- If the grant incorporates animal models, plan on price increases for housing, purchasing, veterinary care, etc.
- If a collaborator is involved, he or she may require a share of the personnel costs as well. (Remember that a senior researcher can be a great asset to a grant, but as he or she tends to have a higher income, this will also mean more share of the grant. A 1-month stipend is often agreeable.)

Once those major costs have been covered, hopefully there is money left for other items, such as equipment needed to conduct the experiment. Just as important as knowing what can be purchased with a budget is knowing what cannot be purchased. For example, smaller grants (ie, institutional and society grants) typically offer a reduced amount of grant money as they do not have the funding available to furnish a lab for a 5-year study. Rather, they expect a return on their investment fairly quickly. In general, this means that a researcher will not be allowed to purchase much (if any) equipment due to the smaller award. Furthermore, some grants have a limit regarding what equipment one can and cannot purchase.

If a researcher is doing cell assays, for example, reagents always seem to end up costing more than one plans for. Budgeting for more than is needed is always a good idea as it is always better to have a little bit of money available for those "what if?" scenarios. Such ancillary study costs can include the following:

- Additional expendable equipment due to accidentally ruined experiments
- Equipment repair
- Software/computers
- Patient stipends and parking

These and other incidental costs are why researchers must think "down the road." Will their department chair provide the additional space needed for these items? Will their lab require 220v freezer plugs? If so, someone will have to pay for electric work. It is important to try to factor these ancillary costs in prior to writing the budget portion of the grant.

So, why is a budget being detailed in a chapter on grant writing? If one is to write a successful grant, every section of the grant must be justified. Specific to the budget, a reviewer who reads a proposal that will go over budget in the first set of experiments will realize very quickly that the author has not thought out the entire process. Just like in life, one must live within his or her budget. If the researcher's budget outline will not allow for completion of the experiment(s), the proposal will end up as a guaranteed rejection. A realistic view (budget) of what is required for the work to be done will help to convince the reviewers that the author of the grant knows how to perform the work proposed in the grant.

Because outlining the budget is so important, one of the first questions that a researcher must ask him- or herself is whether the budget is within reason. To help answer this question, enter the institution's Office of Contracts and Grants. These folks are usually experts in preparing budgets (fill-in spreadsheets are one of the things that make technology tolerable). The initial grant call might be very exciting—$250,000 per year for 5 years. No way a researcher can spend that money, right? Wrong, of course. Just like one's first paycheck is often a lot less than might be hoped for, a grant budget can quickly disappear.

Sidebar 11-11

There is a sort of hierarchy in the research world. If a researcher is at the top of the funding chain, he or she likely has an "established" lab with a lab manager (who may also serve as a tech and scheduler). Those truly at the top of the funding food chain will have a (or multiple) research assistant professor(s), meaning a group of doctorate-level researchers who do most of the lab work but who are not tenure-track. These folks are expensive; the head researcher is likely paying their salary, including fringe (benefits). A bit cheaper than funding research assistant professors are post-doctoral fellows. The NIH is kind enough to dictate their salary based on the number of years they have served as post-doctoral fellows. These folks are more expensive than graduate students, who do not require near the fringe costs but also do not have the detailed experiments nor expertise as do research assistant professors or post-doctoral fellows. Undergraduate students tend to be quite inexpensive, and often do not require salary, but they do require funds.

Salary and Personnel

Most grants will have an entire section devoted to personnel. This section will detail the financial costs related to the individuals involved in the grant, including salary and fringe benefits. Salary is likely one of the highest budget expenses a grant will fund. As discussed earlier, many researchers are on a 9-month appointment, meaning their summer pay—or approximately one-third of their yearly income—must come from somewhere else such as grant funding. For example, a researcher making $70,000 per year on a 9-month contract would need approximately $23,000 from a grant to continue receiving the same monthly paycheck over the summer. However, the final amount must also include fringe benefits (eg, medical, retirement, taxes), so in reality, the cost is even higher. This one area of funding takes a significant bite out of one's budget (Sidebar 11-11).

Most likely, the researcher is not the only one involved in the study. Students, post-doctoral fellows, technicians, and outside support (eg, collaborators) are also all involved and need a salary as well as the associated fringe benefits. Salaries are fixed; therefore, a researcher cannot readjust a salary simply because he or she is running out of money. Although these individuals result in additional budget costs, they are also essential for the success of the grant. If the budget and personnel section does not clearly outline that the researcher and his or her group of experts can do the proposed work, the grant will not be funded. For example, if the researcher is proposing to measure samples via flow cytometry, there should be a section that outlines one of the grant team members' expertise in flow cytometry. If he or she does not have a background that demonstrates proficiency with this technique, the researcher must have someone on the grant who can. If the researcher has difficulty balancing his or her checkbook but the grant requires data analysis using multivariate repeated measures analysis of variance using non-parametric data, it would be best to include on the grant team a brilliant statistician, who is always in demand during grant cycles. A researcher should never "skimp" on essential personnel to save money in the budget because a quality team is needed for the success of most grants applications.

Equipment

Not far behind salaries are the costs of the actual equipment needed to perform the experiments. Biological labs are expensive, as is the equipment needed to properly stock them. Disposables (pipettes, reagents, antibodies) add up in a hurry, so researchers must be sure to budget carefully here. Some exercise-related equipment such as dynamometers can approach $100,000 after price, shipping, and setup fees. While a researcher cannot adjust salary, he or she can request funding for whatever reagents are needed. These equipment costs can be substantial, particularly if using animal models. Mouse housing costs can increase at any time, and not every institution will take pity on funding limitations. Therefore, it is always wise to factor in more costs here than needed. (Researchers should not forget to speak with animal care experts regarding veterinary and husbandry costs, which are sometimes forgotten in budgets.)

Travel

Once the experiments are complete, it does not mean an end to the research project's expenses. In addition to the ongoing salaries, researchers will need to disseminate the findings of their study. This will usually invoke costs relating to travel as well as publication of the results. Specific to travel, researchers will want to show off their data, and they will certainly want to chat with researchers presenting similar work at conferences and workshops, as will their students. This involves costs such as airfare, conference registration fees, hotels, and food, among others. Once having finalized all experiments, the researcher and his or her collaborators will write up the results in a manuscript and submit that manuscript for publication. Some journals are rather expensive to publish in, particularly if figures that require color to be appreciated are required.

Equipment

Each grant will likely have a section devoted to available equipment. While the budget is to be used for equipment that the researcher needs to purchase, the equipment section of a grant will outline that equipment to which the research team has access to for conducting the intricacies of the research project. This section should list not only the equipment in the researcher's lab, but also all equipment that he or she will have access to both on campus (eg, animal care facility) as well as through the other grant collaborators.

The equipment section should not be a bullet list; rather, grant writers should take the time to elaborate on how each relevant piece of equipment has a specific purpose in the grant. This could include physical equipment as well as computer programs, such as those used for data analysis. Detailing each piece of equipment available to the research team will demonstrate that a fully functional lab is available, even if it is not all under one roof. If research is being proposed in which the researcher does not have all of the necessary equipment, he or she needs to establish contact with potential collaborators. For example, if the researcher happens to be near a medical center but works at a smaller institution with limited lab equipment, the researcher will certainly want to (if he or she has not already) speak with people who have this Garden of Eden of scientific instrumentation available to them. It is surprisingly easy to establish contacts and collaborators. Bringing a fundable research idea to a group of scientists whose main role will be to allow that person to do most of the work while they share in the glory of the findings always makes people smile. There are more helpful established researchers out there than one might think; they may even help with the writing of the sections.

Support Letters

If a researcher has a great idea that is potentially fundable, he or she might push that potentially fundable idea into the *definitely* fundable range by including key personnel on the grant, either as a collaborator or as a person of support. Often, there is the "wise old researcher" who has a particular assay, technique, antibody, one-of-a-kind piece of instrumentation, or transgenic model that moves someone's grant from good to great once that person is added to the grant. A letter of support from the individual may go a very long way toward securing funding.

Brain power is one of the best selling points. If this wise old researcher has his or her own PubMed section devoted to his or her scientific advancements, this researcher's benefit as a contributor will be self-evident. Perhaps he or she will not be a direct part of the grant, but the researcher can be someone to whom the PI can turn during the course of the grant work for advice, interpretation, upcoming steps, and alternative hypotheses (meaning the contributing researcher

Sidebar 11-12

Here is a sample letter of support (yes, I did write it for the investigator). Note the emphasis on the need for this particular study as few similar studies existed. Also note how the mentor is spoken of; having a well-established investigator speak highly of the applicant's mentor and establishing a history of successful collaboration will go quite a long way:

To Whom It May Concern:

I am writing this letter of support on behalf of Dr. Thomas Lowder. I have agreed to serve as a co-collaborator for his grant submission proposal entitled "Effects of Exercise Training on Regulatory T Cells in a Murine Model of Asthma." Dr. Lowder's proposed grant will examine the effects that exercise training may have on Regulatory T cell (T_{reg}) expression and function, as well as the effect(s) that exercise may have on these T_{regs} in an asthma model. These proposed experiments are unique in that little data currently exists about how exercise may affect this particular population of T cells. These proposed studies represent a fantastic opportunity for Dr. Lowder to establish a unique line of research. Little if any research currently exists in the peer-reviewed literature examining the effects that exercise training may have on T_{regs}, and no studies currently available have examined exercise training and T_{regs} using a murine model of asthma.

The laboratory work and the generation of data will be performed by Dr. Lowder under the direct supervision of Dr. ---- I have served as a collaborator with Dr. ---- and can attest to the quality of research performed in her lab. My role in this project will consist of aiding Dr. Lowder in the interpretation and analysis of the data generated from these proposed experiments. Further, I will provide consultation for the inevitable questions that arise during the research process. I feel that I am very well-suited to serve as an advisor on this project. With over two decades of experience in researching T cells and cytokines, I have nearly 60 peer-reviewed publications that have examined CD4+ T cells and/or T_{regs}. I currently have several active NIH grants, including two RO1 National Institute of Allergy and Infectious Disease–funded grants examining T cell function and one National Institute of Diabetes and Digestive and Kidney Disease–funded grant that is examining T_{regs}.

I am very excited to be a co-collaborator with Dr. Lowder on this grant proposal. He has impressed me with his unique background and with his knowledge of T_{regs}, a field that is evolving and expanding almost daily. The data that will be generated from these proposed experiments will greatly contribute not only to the field of T_{regs}, but also to those researching asthma, inflammation, and exercise. The funding of this grant will allow for Dr. Lowder to begin a successful record of NIH funding. This will greatly aid in his transition from a post-doctoral fellow to an independent researcher. I fully encourage the funding of this grant.

can help to say something positive when the experiments did not work as they were supposed to). A letter of support will go a long way, particularly if one is a newly-minted scientist and does not have a track record of steady funding yet (Sidebar 11-12).

Revisions, Revisions

Submitting a major grant is in itself a major accomplishment. Once submitted, the waiting game begins specific to whether the grant will be funded. The absolute worst thing that will happen after submitting a grant is that it will not be funded. Researchers should understand that most

Sidebar 11-13

Post-rejection comments to self:

- I understood what I wanted to do. That may have been the problem; the people reading my grant were not me, they did not spend 1 year working on this design nor writing and editing the sections.

- I know what I saw, but I did not translate it well enough to be understood by someone who had not performed these experiments.

- My post-doctoral fellow understood this, but she also did a lot of the work so it made sense to her.

- Next time, I will give this to a colleague to read—someone who knows my work but has not done my work.

grants submitted are not funded; however, this should not keep anyone from applying. Accepted and rejected grants both will receive feedback. If a grant is funded, the comments will be constructive and most likely rewarding. Conversely, if the grant is not funded, those comments can hurt. Comments are usually not a reflection of the PI so much as they are a reflection of why the grant is not yet good enough to warrant funding. The approach to take is to step back after reading the comments and try to figure out the basis for why those comments were made. Odds are there are some very good suggestions in those words of rejection that will move the grant resubmission at least a little further up the ladder (Sidebar 11-13).

So, what is there to do next? Resubmit, of course. NIH grant cycles are every 4 months (October, February, and June, to follow the academic year). Society and foundation grants vary in due dates and frequency. Institutional grants are generally much smaller and are offered usually once per year for a particular grant, and each year may consist of an entirely new set of reviewers. If an NIH grant is at the top of the goals for grants to obtain, the PI should plan every submission around these due dates. While reworking (editing, adding requested data, experiments, etc), the PI can maximize momentum by submitting to some of these smaller foundation or institutional grants, but be careful—receiving funding through, say, a private foundation may keep the PI from submitting that same grant to NIH.

Conclusion

Grant writing can be a tedious and highly detailed process. However, grant writing is essential to maintaining an investigator's research line. While an institution may evaluate a researcher's productivity based on research manuscript output, it is successful grant writing that often determines whether the funding will be available to conduct that very research. Therefore, researchers must spend time understanding the intricacies of grant writing and working to improve their grant-writing skills. As those skills improve, the likelihood of being awarded a grant improves as well, along with the increased research opportunities that come with adequate funding.

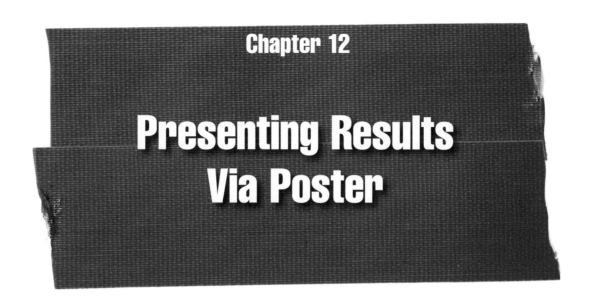

Chapter 12

Presenting Results Via Poster

Sarah A. Manspeaker, PhD, LAT, ATC

Congratulations! Chapter authors at this stage have submitted an abstract of their work that has been accepted for poster presentation at an upcoming venue. Whereas presenting the results of a research project follows many of the same basic section headers as scientific methodology such as Introduction, Methods, Results, etc, the content for display on a poster is quite different. In fact, proper sentence and paragraph structure goes out the door, so to speak. The poster must get its message across in a very brief time frame, so the information must be compact and use pictures and short statements.[1] A poster requires significant streamlining and condensing of information to draw the reader to the highlights of the project. The poster essentially tells the story of the authors' work and can serve as a conversation starter with the audience.[2] This chapter will focus on how to convert ideas from the style used in a scientific paper into the writing style needed for an effective poster, all without losing the content of the message.

Attendees to meetings have limited time to review and browse posters, and they will not spend time on a poster that is not well-structured and aesthetically pleasing. Using proper sentence and paragraph structure is difficult to maintain and likely to not entice a reader when it comes to presenting one's work via poster. Long paragraphs and technical writing are replaced with bullet points, charts, and simplified graphics for ease of information digestion.[3,4] Sports medicine–based examples and sample problems in this chapter will focus on converting an effective sentence into a meaningful bullet point, and recognizing which points presented in a paragraph should be extracted for a poster.

Early Considerations of the Poster

Purpose of the Poster

Once a project author's abstract has been accepted, it is time to determine the direction the poster presentation will take. Thoughtful consideration about the poster's purpose at the event

Knoblauch M. *Professional Writing in Kinesiology and Sports Medicine* (pp 127-148).
© 2019 Taylor & Francis Group.

will be necessary. How does an author intend to communicate the story of his or her work to the audience? Who will be the target audience? Are viewers likely to be specialists in the poster's topic area; representative of multiple disciplines; a mix of the 2? In general, the direction for the poster including what is communicated from the author's viewpoint vs that of the reader needs to occur. Depending on the answer to these questions, the poster's overall design, layout, and selected illustrations may be influenced.

Construction of the Poster

Most posters are constructed utilizing a single slide in Microsoft PowerPoint, though other programs may be used if the target poster size warrants and/or the author has the software available and knows how to use it. Other options include Microsoft Publisher, Canvas (Instructure), CorelDRAW (Corel), Adobe Illustrator or InDesign (Adobe Systems), or online templates available for download. Spending time reviewing the requirements of the presentation will allow the authors to identify which design program will be best for the intended product.

Layout of the Poster

Another important aspect to consider in poster construction is the formatting requirements set forth by the entity (ie, conference, symposium, organization, etc) to which the poster will be presented. As mentioned previously, the initial layout, design, and format must be intentionally selected based on the audience and purposefully targeted to those who will be exposed to the poster.[5] However, more physical, structure-based consideration of the specific requirements of the entity must also be incorporated. For example, there may be specific dimension restrictions on height and width, abstract requirements, headers, or graphics limitations that might be set forth by the entity. Typical poster dimensions are 44 inches (112 cm) high by 68 inches (173 cm) wide. Upon acceptance of the poster, the author will typically receive an email containing specific guidelines or a weblink to requirements. It is vital to check all communications from the entity to determine what the official poster requirements might be. It is also important to note that these requirements may change from year to year, so relying on a sample or template that is outdated may not yield the best results. Table 12-1 features recent poster requirements for both the American College of Sports Medicine (ACSM)[6] and the National Athletic Trainers' Association.[7]

Once the key content focus of the poster and the guidelines to be followed have been determined, specific thought regarding the spacing and layout options come into play. Visual cues[8] can play an important role in guiding eye gaze. The visual components provided on the poster will be very important to the overall design. Specifically, authors should include tables, photographs, or figures that will serve as visual cues for where the viewer should look next.[8] The final poster will feature a combination of text, graphics, and/or tables. Ultimately, the goal is to arrange the content so that the larger, more aesthetic parts of the poster draw the most attention.

In consideration of this visual cueing, authors should be aware of how the eye scans surroundings and should construct the poster accordingly. Typically, the reader will first read in a horizontal direction across the upper content.[9] Next, the reader will visually scroll down the page, reading across in the same horizontal direction, covering a shorter area than the upper section. As the poster is viewed, the reader's brain will most likely try to identify central shapes within the poster.[8] Rectangles[10] and triangles, for example, are intriguing shapes to the human eye and, as such, authors may choose to format their poster around these centralized ideas. Given that the poster itself will likely be a rectangle, the eye-brain will scan the poster in a Z- or F-pattern (Figure 12-1). The Z-pattern may be beneficial in allowing for all important information to be viewed, so highlighting the most important pieces of information in this pattern may help to further focus the reader's attention as desired. As the eye scans horizontally, authors can separate the material into vertical sections on the poster that can then be read in a repeated horizontal fashion.

Table 12-1. Sample Poster Guidelines From National Organizations		
	AMERICAN COLLEGE OF SPORTS MEDICINE	**NATIONAL ATHLETIC TRAINERS' ASSOCIATION**
DIMENSIONS	Fit within 4 feet high by 8 feet wide	44 inches high by 68 inches wide
REQUIRED CONTENT	Abstract (upper left corner)	N/A
TYPICAL CONTENT	Introduction Experimental design Methods Results Tables/figures/graphs Summary and conclusion Acknowledgment	Abstract Purpose Methods Results Implications Etc
FONT SIZE	View from 3 feet away Suggested: • Times font in 18-point • 11 characters and spaces per horizontal inch • 4 lines per vertical inch	View from 4 feet away
TABLES/GRAPHS	High resolution	High resolution
SECURING METHOD	Push pins	Push pins

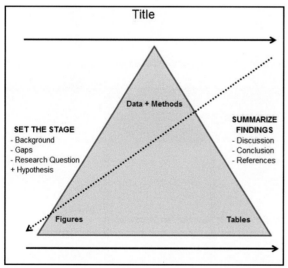

Figure 12-1. Format for eye scanning consideration.

This repeated horizontal structure will allow the viewer to easily read from left to right across the poster.[10] Regarding the F-pattern of viewing, readers may lose or skip over some information if the left side of the poster is overloaded. Figures 12-2 through 12-4 and Poster 12-1 portray sample layouts that may be appropriate for consideration.

Figure 12-2. Sample dual-column layout for more textual heavy content balanced with illustrations.

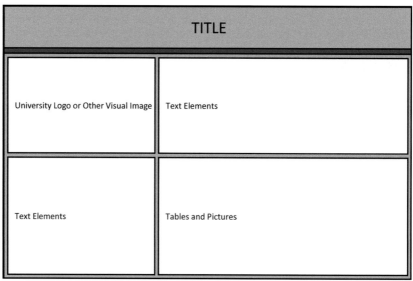

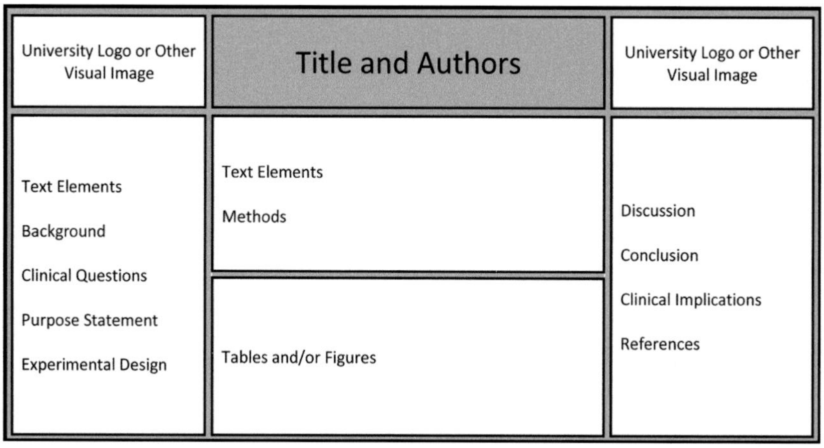

Figure 12-3. Sample triple-column layout for combined text and tables/figures.

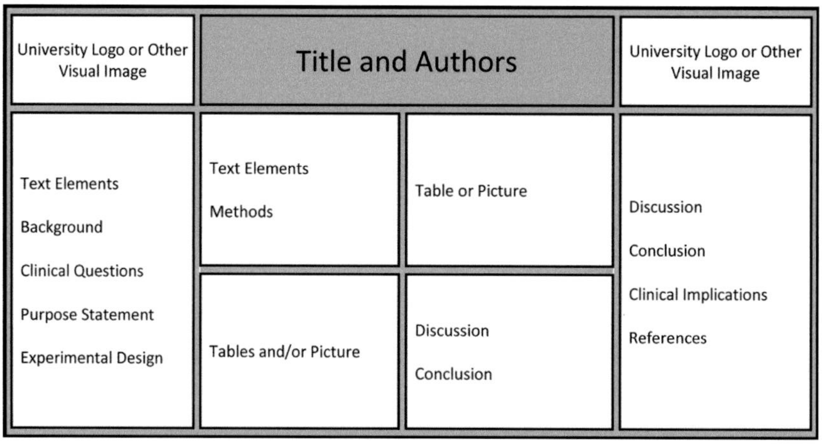

Figure 12-4. Sample quadruple-column layout for a mix of text and illustrative information.

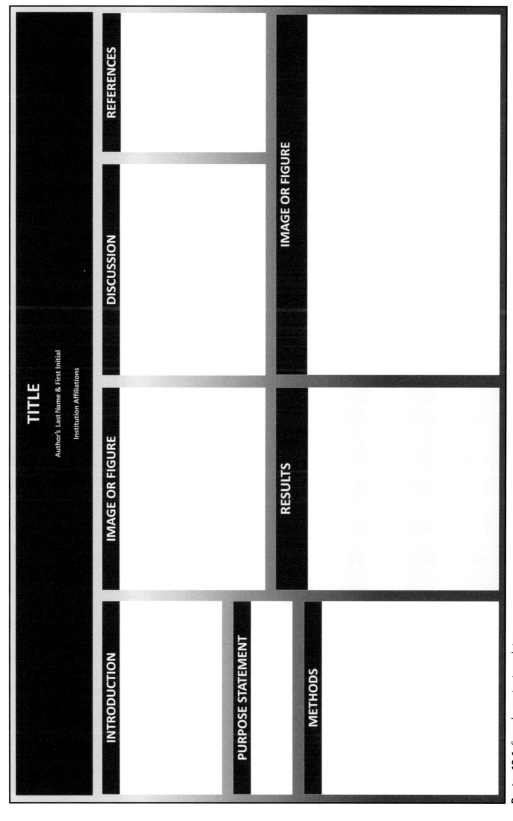

Poster 12-1. Sample poster template.

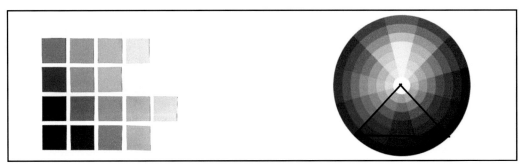

Figure 12-5. Color scheme options: monochromatic and full color wheel with 3 adjacent colors that could complement each other in poster design.

Templates and Color Guides

When an author begins assembling the poster, he or she should inquire about whether his or her school or employer has a template that should be followed. If there is in fact a template, it is suggested to use it, but know that it is adaptable (in most cases). Regarding the background, authors should weigh the options of a full-color background vs the aforementioned boxes for content. Color gets attention; it should be used wisely and to the author's advantage. A crisp, light-colored background, with dark font color for text typically shows up well in most rooms. Authors should be careful to not overdo the color or mix too many colors; for example, choosing one monochromatic color scheme (Poster 12-2) but using a variety of shades within that scheme may be beneficial. Additionally, use of adjacent colors in a color wheel may help to achieve this appearance[11]; Figure 12-5 provides an example of how to identify adjacent colors in a color wheel. Incorporation of contrasting shades to compliment the background color and graphics will help to emphasize key points and significant findings; the goal is to achieve a balance of colors that will hold attention and not distract from the poster.[11,12] Tables, figures, and photos should all align well with other color aspects of the poster. Additionally, the author's institution may provide requirements for appropriate and acceptable color palates for their formats. Generally, authors are encouraged to avoid a dark background with white font as this often results in the words blending together and appear as one large block from a distance rather than distinct words. While large font size can help prevent blending from occurring, it is better to just avoid that color scheme in the first place.

Regarding font size, generally the font should be easily read from approximately 4 feet away. Titles should be a minimum of 40-point font type with the remaining text being within the range of around 24-point font.[4] These font sizes are suggestions and may be increased as necessary, keeping in mind that larger text decreases the amount of information that can be provided. Additional consideration should be given to use font types that will enhance readability. Sans serif fonts (see Chapter 13) may be considered for titles and headers (ie, Verdana, Helvetica), while serif fonts such as Times New Roman may be useful in areas with larger amounts of text.[11] In general, authors should be judicious in their selection of what information to present as this will provide a framework for the poster, thus allowing them to work backward to determine font type and size based on information presented and space available.

When considering logos and graphics, authors should be aware that a university, research lab, or other entity may have restrictions on what illustrations/logotypes can be utilized. Many universities will have a specific set of graphic standards that must be followed when utilizing their logo. Specific investigation into color schemes, shadowing, or manipulation of logos should be sought in advance. In general, it is best to ask the entity what approved logos exist and what permissions must be attained to use them. It is also important to note that university guidelines often will provide incorrect uses of the logo that can help guide authors to correct inclusion of graphics. It is not appropriate to locate a photo or logo on the internet and embed it within the poster; rather, all information must be cited appropriately and attribute credit for the illustration as appropriate.

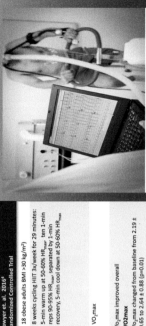

Poster 12-2. Monochromatic sample. (Reprinted with permission from Dr. Sarah A. Manspeaker, PhD, LAT, ATC.)

Poster 12-3. Contrast color with approved logo example. (Reprinted with permission from Dr. Erica Beidler, PhD, ATC.)

Poster 12-3 serves as a good example of logos that are approved for use by Duquesne University and Michigan State University. Both logos are featured prominently and appropriately in respective corners, in color combinations that are appropriate to both institutions.

Sidebar 12-1

Benefits of bullet points:

- Draw the reader to important information that you have selected
- Allow for quick identification of key facts and statements
- Work well if the first words are of the same part of speech and are similar in length

For poster construction in general, following the guidelines provided in this section will be beneficial, though it is worth noting that creation of a unique poster is also of importance. Poster authors typically have the creative license to customize certain items such as border, background color(s), layout, etc. Though a template can be followed, personalizing the template to an author's individual style while enhancing the reader's interpretation of the material will help create a well-rounded product.

Grammatical Structure

Trying to fit properly formatted sentences into a poster results in information overload that either requires microscopic font or requires so much text that the reader is psychologically exhausted after reading just the poster's introduction. A paragraph structure may be intimidating to the reader's eye; thus, bullet points are acceptable and encouraged to highlight the most important topics in a structured format. Bullet points are commonly displayed as short series of text in a list or series that are demarcated by a circle, check, or other symbol to serve as the "bullet." Bullet points may still be structured as full sentences following the bullet, but they may also feature significant truncation of sentences. There are several benefits to including bullet points instead of full sentences on a poster as bulleted in Sidebar 12-1. In the interest of keeping a reader's attention, poster authors will want to avoid large blocks of continuous, sentence-based text; these types of structures are difficult for the readers to follow on a poster and will most likely lose their interest. Posters should have minimal text, which, in turn, allows for larger font size and incorporation of more graphics/figures. The more text that is included, the less room there is for highlighting one's results. With each of these points in mind, condensing the language as much as possible is essential.

While condensing information is important, acronyms may be used, but they should only be those that are commonly known among the population to which the author is presenting. If presenting to a group outside of the author's normal population, it is typically not recommended to use acronyms. A general rule may be for authors to write their text on the poster, read it, condense it, read it again, and condense it again. Rarely will the first edition of the writing be succinct enough.

Another facet to consider when designing a poster is the attention-drawing nature of the design. Poster authors should not design their posters with the simple goal of standing in front of it—it is a poster, not a chandelier; make it approachable. Layouts, illustrations, and textual modifications that allow for the drawing of attention during the poster's presentation should be considered. The reader should be able to quickly identify important facts and information. For example, authors might consider what points on a graph can be highlighted by using **bold** or CAPITALIZED text, underlining, or *italicization*; the more an author emphasizes points on the poster, the more the audience will also recognize these facets. The bottom line is to include and highlight information on the poster that is worth identifying and interacting with (Table 12-2).[3]

In summary, the primary goal is to create a poster that meets the requirements of the entity at which an author will be presenting, while providing relevant content from his or her work. Authors should be sure to review samples of what has been done previously in related topics or at their

Table 12-2. Tips for Maximizing Information and Viewing of the Poster

1. Include the most important information at the top of each section of the poster.
2. Use headings wisely, and be sure they stand out from other text so viewers can interpret them quickly.
3. Be sure headings are specific key words related to the project; these may include traditional abstract headings or others that are unique to the information.
4. Group related information together so it stands out: use either boxes, borders, variations in background color, etc.
5. **Bold** key words and statements.
6. Use bullet points and/or numbering to narrow focus to a list or process.
7. Do not be afraid to cut unnecessary content to reduce clutter and text.

Adapted from Pernice K. F-shaped pattern of reading on the web: misunderstood, but still relevant (even on mobile). Nielsen Norman Group Web site. Available at: https://www.nngroup.com/articles/f-shaped-pattern-reading-web-content. Published November 12, 2017. Accessed March 1, 2018.

Table 12-3. Anticipated Process for Construction of a Research Poster	
PREPARATION	Select key points from the project to convey to the audience.
	Determine appropriate content.
	Determine poster construction requirements.
CREATION	Establish desired design/layout.
	Construct the poster with content according to design/layout.
PROOF AND POLISH	Review content, layout, and aesthetics.
	Print a sample on smaller paper, and evaluate for details.
	Review and revise accordingly.
FINAL PRODUCT	Print.
	Present.

respective institution. For example, what was the general structure? What aspects of the poster caught the authors' eye? What aspects were easy or hard to follow? How might those areas influence structure and layout of the author's poster? Keep in mind that it is not necessary to recreate the wheel during poster construction, but rather make it unique to one's own work and the key findings. Table 12-3 features a general overview of the process authors can anticipate undertaking for successful design of the research poster.

Presenting Information Via Graphics

Posters allow the author to present their work with a combination of text and visual data.[13] Tables, charts, graphs, and other visual images can be great ways to tell the story of your work and present the results and/or other important content.[5,13,14] Creating simple charts (eg, Microsoft SmartArt, Microsoft Excel, etc) that highlight specific results, including significance values and point estimates, can help the reader view effects and interactions. Charts may also help to illustrate variables of interest, confidence intervals, or other relevant data points in a quick and digestible manner.[1] It is important to note that formatting changes may be necessary if a chart has been constructed in a software program other than where the poster is being constructed. Regardless, the author must keep in mind that charts should have clear titles on all axes, minimal or no grid lines that may distract the eye away from significant plot points, easily identifiable plot lines, a legend (where applicable), and a concise title.[11]

Anecdotally, some authors prefer to use more images and less text on a poster to enhance the storytelling ability of the poster, thus increasing the chance of favorable reading by the audience. Generally, authors should aim to provide types of images that are familiar to the audience in an appropriate number. Each visual image should be provided in conjunction with a title that describes the content of the chart. Poster 12-2 illustrates a successful infusion of charts and tables.

Adding Content to the Poster

The Abstract as a Guide to Poster Construction

While an abstract is a brief summary of a research project that allows a reader to quickly determine the purpose of the work, it is designed to provide a great amount of detail in the least amount of words. Where a poster is often accepted based on the submitted abstract, it is not ideal to simply copy and paste the abstract into the appropriate headings on a poster. This approach will likely leave the reader unclear about the full scope of the project and wanting more information. As listed in the ACSM guidelines (see Table 12-1),[6] an abstract is required for their poster presentations. This requirement is not universal and should always be supplemented by additional information in other sections. What a reader will often see in poster presentations is a pasted abstract in small font, while all other sections are outlined in bullet-point fashion, trying to make room for the abstract. This structure violates many recommendations made previously in this chapter regarding font size, aesthetics, and overall construction.

When constructing the poster, it is best to keep the abstract as a reference guide for the flow of information, but give each section its own individual attention and emphasis. Keep in mind that readers will have varying levels of experience with the author's topic; some people may be content experts but not well-versed in methodology while others will be methods experts but not know much about the specific topic.[4] The bottom line is the poster author is the expert on the methods and the content; therefore, it is vital that the author provide enough content for both the topic and the methodology to clearly convey all aspects of the research completed.

In general, the poster should be designed around 2 to 3 main findings.[3,5] Identify what key pieces of information should be conveyed to the viewer (ie, take-home points) and design the title, text, and supplemental tables/figures around these points, keeping the poster as simple and concise as possible.[3,5] If an author is having a difficult time succinctly putting something into words, consider whether a photograph or figure might better illustrate the point.[4] Table 12-3 provides suggested tips for construction of a poster. Further information for each of these sections will be provided later in the chapter.

Title

At the top of each poster should be a centered title of less than 16 words. It is best to keep the title simple and directly related to the project findings; in other words, it is a variation of the main message of the research.[2] One consideration should be regarding whether the title relates only to the research question or reveals a direction of the findings as well. That decision is up to the authors, but anecdotally, some researchers find it more enticing for readers to not know the result of a study simply by reading the title. Once the succinct title has been selected, it is best to include it in a font size at 40 points or larger.[4] Following the title, all authors should be listed in order and reflect the order of contribution to the research study (see Chapter 14 for more information on author order).

Figure 12-6. Sample title section of poster.

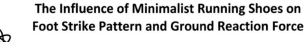

**The Influence of Minimalist Running Shoes on
Foot Strike Pattern and Ground Reaction Force**

Author FA, Contributor SE, Backer DP

Presentation University, Harrisburg, PA

All required information for the presenting entity should be provided and may include, though is not limited to, last name, first initial(s), and workplace affiliation. Any institutional requirements such as logos or branding items should be positioned to offset the title appropriately. Figure 12-6 provides a sample of a well-constructed title section.

Introduction and Purpose Statement

For the Introduction or Background section, it is often recommended to briefly summarize pertinent background information that helps to establish the relevance of the author's work. Ideally, this section will be between 2 to 4 sentences or bullet points and should include the purpose and/or scientific aims of the study. If relevant, the hypothesis may be identified here as well. It is important to consider what information the viewer must have in order to understand the "story" of the poster. If a statement is deemed irrelevant to the story, it should be omitted from the poster. For factual information in this section, citations that link the reader to the reference section of the poster should be provided. While superscript references may be helpful in creating more space, the format should match the presentation guidelines appropriately. Oftentimes, this section of the poster contains the most references.

Another key component of the poster is the purpose statement and/or clinical question. This statement should be clear and stand out on the poster. Poster authors may see this statement embedded within the introduction, or it may have its own standalone location on the poster. Ultimately, the poster's layout should draw the reader's eye to this statement via the use of bold or colored font, strategic location on the page, or some other mechanism. Furthermore, authors should limit the purpose statement to one sentence whenever possible. An exception to this general rule would be when there are secondary study aims. A sample introduction that is structured utilizing bullet points and highlights the purpose statement in bold is provided in Table 12-4. For work that is centered around a clinical question in PICO (patient, intervention, comparison, outcome) format, this information should be clearly identified as such in addition to the clinical question.

Methods

The goal of the Methods section of the poster is to provide a succinct summary of the process undertaken during the research phase.[3] An overly detailed description of the methods utilized may diminish the value of other portions of the presentation. The author's aim is to provide enough information to follow the storyline of the project but not overcrowd the poster with too much detail. Keep in mind that the reader will likely be interested in the introduction/background/rationale, results, and relevance of the results. The methods are unlikely to be considered the reader's primary area of interest. While most methods sections will be very succinct and to the point, such as a web-based survey needing only 1 to 2 sentences to describe the methods, other research types may require a more detailed description (Table 12-5). For example, a poster of a critically appraised topic or systematic review will require an author to provide much more detail, such as the terms utilized during the search strategy (Table 12-6). Additionally, critically appraised topic and systematic review methodologies will need to also state the sources utilized for the literature search, inclusion and exclusion criteria, as well as levels of included evidence with

Table 12-4. Sample Introduction and Purpose Statements

SAMPLE INTRODUCTION USING BULLET POINTS WITH PURPOSE STATEMENT EMBEDDED	SAMPLE INTRODUCTION USING SENTENCE STRUCTURE AND A SEPARATE BOX FOR PURPOSE STATEMENT
• Interprofessional Education (IPE) provides a background for practitioners to collaborate with multiple health care professionals with the goal of improving the overall communication and ultimately enhancing patient outcomes.[1] • IPE aims to address competencies within 4 domains: 1) roles and responsibilities; 2) teams and teamwork; 3) communication; and 4) values and ethics.[2] • Compared to the other domains, the values and ethics domain is less frequently described in published studies examining the effectiveness of IPE. • The purpose of this study was to examine health science student perceptions of an IPE Ethics Workshop.	Exertional Rhabdomyolysis is the breakdown of skeletal muscle tissue following intense physical activity that results in impairment of the cell membrane, which allows intracellular contents to be released into the bloodstream. Diagnosis of Exertional Rhabdomyolysis (ER) among athletes has increased over the past 15 years, yet conclusive information regarding diagnosis, treatment, and return to activity is lacking. This study aims to synthesize the available evidence regarding Creatine Kinase (CK) levels at diagnosis, types of treatment, length of hospital stay, and return to activity. **Clinical Question:** Among athletes, is fluid resuscitation or nutritional intervention more effective in treating Exertional Rhabdomyolysis?

Table 12-5. Experimental Design Methods Section Comparison

TEXT-HEAVY METHODS SECTION	SUCCINCT METHODS SECTION
A 1x2 repeated measures non-randomized experimental design was used to study the effects of diathermy and thermal therapeutic ultrasound on hip flexion range of motion (ROM). The independent variable was the hip flexion ROM at different intervals pre- and post-treatment. Twenty-two healthy college students aged between 19 and 25 participated in this study. The participants had no history of any significant lower leg injuries. Participants' bilateral hip flexion ROM was evaluated by a Certified Athletic Trainer prior to treatment through goniometric measurement techniques. Then, the participants received diathermy @ 48 W continuous for 15 minutes on 1 hamstring group and thermal ultrasound @ 3.3 MHz 1.5 W/cm^2 for 7 minutes to the other hamstring group. Following the treatments, hip flexion ROM was reassessed at the following intervals: immediately following treatment, 2 minutes, 5 minutes, and 10 minutes post-treatment.	A 1x2 repeated measures design evaluating diathermy in comparison to thermal ultrasound on hip flexion range of motion was conducted on college students (n = 22, 19-25 y/o) with no history of lower leg injury performed hip flexion range of motion as measured by a goniometer.

Table 12-6. Systematic Review Methods Section Comparison

TEXT-HEAVY METHODS SECTION	SUCCINCT METHODS SECTION
Search strategy: A comprehensive search of the following databases with no date limitation was conducted: CINAHL, ProQuest, Embase, SPORTDiscus, PubMed, Physical Education Index, and the Joanna Briggs Institute Database of Systematic Reviews & Implementation Reports. Results were limited to those available in English. Methodological quality: Two independent reviewers evaluated the retrieved papers for methodological quality using the standardized critical appraisal instruments from the Joanna Briggs Institute Meta-Analysis of Statistics and Review Instruments (JBI-MAStARI). Data collection: Data was extracted from the papers by 2 independent reviewers using the standardized JBI extraction tool.	• Quantitative review of studies including athletes 15 years old and older • Databases searched: CINAHL, ProQuest, Embase, SPORTDiscus, PubMed, Physical Education Index • 14 studies were included in the final review for a total of 53 athletes (50 males, 3 females, age 21 ± 3.79) • Descriptive statistics were calculated for all pertinent variables; however, all variables were not present in all studies • Pearson product-moment correlation was computed to assess the relationship between the CK levels at admission and days of hospitalization and between length of hospital stay and time to return to activity

Clinical Question: Among athletes, is fluid resuscitation/replacement or nutritional intervention more effective in treating Exertional Rhabdomyolysis?

justification. When creating this content, authors should be sure to present the search process in its logical order and that the poster provides all relevant information including the 5 Ws: who, what, where, when, and how of data collection.[4]

Results

The results section should effectively present the most important findings of the study. The goal of presenting results in a poster should be to highlight the main findings that are of primary interest to the reader. Most often, it is best to present the top 2 to 3 key results and have them already translated into a style fitting for the poster (ie, in a reader-friendly format that may include tables, charts, or bullet points rather than full sentence statements).[4,5] In general, poster authors should be as clear and succinct as possible in the presentation of their information.

When designing the poster, authors should consider what visuals can be used in the results section to draw in the viewer. Any selected graphics should be of high resolution and clearly labeled for ease of viewing and interpretation. For statistical items, it is best for confidence intervals, point estimates, and statistical significance to be easily identified on the graphics.[4] Additionally, all graphics must have a title that is both easily read and provides a thorough description of the graphic content.

Further consideration should be given to the location of the results in reference to the remainder of the poster. Results do not often make sense on the far left or right side of the poster. Rather, it is suggested to place results in the middle section of the poster to better draw the reader's eye; this layout will also permit for the background and discussion information to be presented on the sides. Poster 12-4 depicts the results presented in this manner. Authors should keep in mind that they will likely be referring to their results a lot when presenting and, therefore, should be confident in interacting with this section.

Poster 12-4. Simplified layout with results chart. (Reprinted with permission from Dr. Laura Kunkel, EdD, LAT, ATC, PES.)

Table 12-7. Sample of Condensed Results	
FULL TEXT OPTION	**BULLET POINT OPTION**
Participants identified perceived barriers to the use of evidence-based practice in clinical practice. These responses and thematic trends were consistently identified in the areas of *time, accessibility of evidence, knowledge related to* evidence-based practice, *applicability of evidence,* and *the culture of their practice environment.*	• Time • Accessibility of evidence • Knowledge related to evidence-based practice • Applicability of evidence • Culture of practice environment

When authors present the results section on their poster, succinctly providing key information will be vital. The sample in Table 12-7 provides a text-heavy description of qualitative results of a study, specifically the themes related to barriers to use of evidence-based practice. This textual description is then truncated significantly into bullet points. As shown in the example, the use of bullet points decreases the needed space and more easily highlights the qualitative results of the study. Poster 12-5 depicts a sample of a 2-column layout with well-presented qualitative results from a project.

Discussion

Similar to the other sections of the poster, only the most relevant information should be included in the discussion, and that information should be presented in a concise manner on the poster. In essence, the discussion should close the loop on the introduction and results while providing an "answer" to the author's purpose statement/clinical question. Given the likelihood that the discussion will convey clinical relevance to the audience, this is a place where the author can offer expanded information if the space is available. Poster authors must ensure that all statements are unique in that they do not simply repeat the results and do not attempt to overstate the significance of the findings. Keep the points simple and relevant.

References and Additional Information

Given the factual and scientific-based nature of the research poster, references are often used in high quantity and are a must for inclusion on the poster so the reader can seek additional information if desired. Depending on space, consider which references are considered key elements of the poster. While it would be ideal to provide all references utilized for the full project, space may not permit this information. There may likely only be room for 3 to 5 references on the poster; therefore, authors must make them count. For example, a generalized statement in the introduction section may not need to be provided on the poster. However, if a statement reads as factual and an author is presenting to an audience unfamiliar with his or her terminology, it is likely best to cite the information. It should also be noted that the entity where the presentation is being given may have requirements for reference formatting, and these should be followed diligently.

If an author finds that his or her poster lacks the space to fit all references, or other information such as results outside of the primary findings, he or she may consider providing viewers with additional resources to learn more about the project. Such mechanisms may include providing a handout below the poster board or use of a quick response (QR) code. Inclusion of a QR code allows the reader to use a smart phone to access additional resources relevant to the author's work. Specific information authors may wish to refer readers to could include the full reference list, a

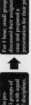
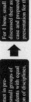
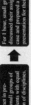
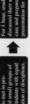
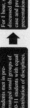

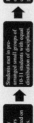

Poster 12-5. Qualitative results. (Reprinted with permission from Caryssa McCool.)

> ### Sidebar 12-2
>
> Specific questions to ask the printer:
>
> 1. What are the material options for printing? Options may include matte finish paper, high gloss paper, cotton, etc.
> 2. What is the cost for the poster size needed as well as for the type of material selected?
> 3. By what format should the poster be delivered to the printer? Email attachment? In-person delivery via thumb drive? Other?
> 4. What is the turn-around time on printing? How far in advance must it be there in order to have an on-time delivery to the author?
> 5. Is there a specific type of program or computer software program preferred for construction?

link to a laboratory website, further contact information for the investigators, video files that highlight portions of methodology, additional readings etc. Poster 12-6 provides an example of a text-heavy poster where the authors may have considered condensing content and utilizing additional resources to convey the desired amount of information.

Affiliations and Acknowledgements

It is important to recognize those that made significant contribution to the author's work when appropriate. Such recognition may be given to individuals that provided insight on the project itself or assisted with poster design. Additional consideration may be given to recognize funding sources that may be relevant for disclosure. Depending on the level of importance and contribution, if space permits, these affiliations and acknowledgements should be included.

Content Consideration: Too Much Empty Space

After telling the short story of their project, authors may find that they have a decent amount of empty space on the poster. There are some general suggestions that may be evaluated to fill that space appropriately. Quick considerations may include adding an image or 2 that are related to the work or adjusting the font size. If those options do not satisfy the space, adjustments to the overall layout of the poster, such as expanding or shortening column widths, increasing header or title size, etc may work.

Printing Considerations

When beginning poster construction, it is important for authors to look ahead to where the poster will be printed. Knowing this information in advance will help the author design the poster according the printer's specifications and determine the timeline needed to have the poster in his or her possession in time for the presentation.

The struggle is real when considering the formatting issues between a MAC and personal computer during poster construction. Authors should check with their poster's printer regarding the preferred program for constructing the poster (Sidebar 12-2). As one might imagine, it is a terrible moment when an author goes to print his or her poster only to find out that the poster is not displaying properly on the computer or printer that is being used (Sidebar 12-3).

UNIVERSITY APPROVED LOGO

The Efficacy of Two Thermal Modalities on Hip Flexion

UNIVERSITY APPROVED LOGO

Author FN, Secondus MN, Contributors PD

Sport Science Research Laboratory, Contributing University, Citytown, USA

Abstract

Proper extensibility of the human body's musculature is important for the reduction of injuries. The hamstring muscle group is especially important when discussing flexibility since even a slight decrease can be detrimental to an athlete's performance. Previous research has demonstrated the efficacy of thermal modalities especially diathermy and therapeutic ultrasound to provide immediate increases in range of motion. However, there is a gap in the literature comparing the effectiveness of these two modality treatments on large muscle groups.

PURPOSE:
To investigate the relationship between the use of diathermy and thermal ultrasound modality treatments and the effects on hamstring flexibility range of motion (ROM) in healthy college-aged participants.

METHODS:
Twenty-two healthy college students aged between 19 and 25 participated in this study. The participants had no history of any significant lower leg injuries. Participants' bi-lateral hip flexion ROM was evaluated by a Certified Athletic Trainer prior to treatment through goniometric measurement techniques. Then, the participants received diathermy @ 48 W continuous for 15 minutes on one hamstring group and thermal ultrasound @ 3.3 Mhz 1.5 W/cm2 for 7 minutes to the other hamstring group. Following the treatments, hip flexion ROM was re-assessed at the following intervals: immediately following treatment, 2 minutes, 5 minutes and 10 minutes post treatment.

RESULTS:
The effects of diathermy and thermal ultrasound were analyzed utilizing a two-way analysis of variance (time x groups) indicated a significant relationship of time. Mauchly's sphericity was significant at the $p<.05$ level therefore Huynh-Felt correction was utilized. $F(3.553,149.232)= 9.100$ $p<=.000$. However, there was no significance between the type of treatment $F(3.553, 149.232) = .574$ $p = .661$

CONCLUSION:
Results demonstrated that the use of both thermal ultrasound and shortwave diathermy produced a statistically significant effect on hamstring flexibility ROM over a period time. Specifically regardless of treatment intervention, the results suggested that flexibility exercise should be initiated immediately up to 2 minutes following the modality treatment for maximal benefit.

Introduction

Proper extensibility of the human body's musculature is important for the reduction of injuries. The hamstring muscle group is especially important when discussing flexibility since even a slight decrease can be detrimental to an athlete's performance. Increasing the core temperature above four degrees Celsius will increase collagen tissue extensibility and decrease tissue viscosity (Draper, et al., 2002). High intensity pulsed shortwave diathermy can heat areas vigorously, inducing muscle relaxation and reducing muscles spasms and joint stiffness. These two deep heating modalities can provide immediate increases in range of motion. The use of diathermy should be more effective than ultrasound since the hamstrings are large and it can increase temperature in larger areas, but research shows very minute benefits (Draper, et al., 2002). Studies completed by Ahmed, et al., (2014) and Akbari, et al., (2006) resulted in increased range of motion within the hamstrings due to ultrasound usage combined with stretching. However, there is a gap in the literature comparing the effectiveness of these two modality treatments on large muscle groups.

Methods

Subjects: Twenty-two healthy subjects (11 Males & 19 Females) with no known hamstring injuries at the time of the intervention, no history of knee or hip surgeries in the last year and no documented participation in a hamstring or quadriceps rehabilitation program within the last six months volunteered for this study. All subjects provided written informed consent; this study was approved by the University institutional review board.

Design: A 1x2 repeated measures non-randomized experimental design was used to study the effects of diathermy and thermal therapeutic ultrasound on hip flexion range of motion (ROM). The independent variable was the hip flexion ROM at different intervals pre and post treatment. The dependent variables for each measure of ROM were the diathermy treatment and the thermal therapeutic ultrasound.

Methods: The participants were supine and a certified athletic trainer (ATC) passively moved the participants ' hip into flexion and stopped when he received maximal hip flexion of the participants noted to stop. An initial goniometry measurement was taken (Fig.2) according to contemporary practice alignment and protocols. Following the initial measurements of each hip, the treatments were applied simultaneously to the two distal hamstrings. The participants remained prone in the treatment with the lower extremity fully supported by the treatment table. The are was properly prepped for ultrasound with an alcohol pad and then conductive gel was placed on the treatment area. One ATC performed a Diathermy treatment on one leg while the thermal ultrasound treatment was completed on the other leg; 8 minutes later to ensure both treatments ended simultaneously.

The following diathermy parameters were used based on the most current evidenced-based research and the Auto Therm 395 Shortwave Diathermy® unit was set to 800 microsecond bust duration, 800 bursts per second, 800 microsecond interburst interval, and root mean output average of 48 W. The Chattanooga Intelect® Legend XT Thermal Ultrasound treatment followed the following parameters: 3 MHz, 1.5 W/cm2, for 7 minutes.

Following the completion of each individual treatment that ended simultaneously, the participants' hip flexion ROM was evaluated immediately following treatment and again at the following intervals: post-treatment 2minutes, post-treatment 5 minutes and post treatment 10 minutes with the same ATC conducting the initial hip flexion ROM measurements utilizing contemporary goniometry hip flexion ROM protocols.

Measure: ROM

Group	Time	Mean	Std. Error	95% Confidence Interval Lower Bound	95% Confidence Interval Upper Bound
1	1	93.455	2.141	89.134	97.776
	2	96.045	2.143	91.720	100.370
	3	95.000	1.868	91.230	98.770
	4	94.364	1.672	90.989	97.738
	5	92.727	1.816	89.062	96.392
2	1	92.864	2.141	88.543	97.185
	2	97.045	2.143	92.720	101.370
	3	96.364	1.868	92.593	100.134
	4	95.136	1.672	91.762	98.511
	5	93.682	1.816	90.017	97.347

Mauchly's Test of Sphericity[a]

Measure: ROM

Within Subjects Effect	Mauchly's W	Approx. Chi-Square	df	Sig.	Epsilon[b] Greenhouse-Geisser	Epsilon[b] Huynh-Feldt	Epsilon[b] Lower-bound
Time	.521	26.968	9	.001	.795	.865	.250

Tests of Within-Subjects Effects

Measure: ROM

Source		Type III Sum of Squares	df	Mean Square	F	Sig.	Partial Eta Squared
Time	Sphericity Assumed	395.027	4	98.757	9.100	.000	.178
	Greenhouse-Geisser	395.027	3.180	124.212	9.100	.000	.178
	Huynh-Feldt	395.027	3.553	111.177	9.100	.000	.178
	Lower-bound	395.027	1.000	395.027	9.100	.004	.178
Time * Group	Sphericity Assumed	24.936	4	6.234	.574	.682	.013
	Greenhouse-Geisser	24.936	3.180	7.841	.574	.643	.013
	Huynh-Feldt	24.936	3.553	7.018	.574	.661	.013
	Lower-bound	24.936	1.000	24.936	.574	.453	.013
Error (Time)	Sphericity Assumed	1823.236	168	10.853			
	Greenhouse-Geisser	1823.236	133.572	13.650			
	Huynh-Feldt	1823.236	149.232	12.217			
	Lower-bound	1823.236	42.000	43.410			

Results

The effects of diathermy and thermal ultrasound were analyzed utilizing a two-way analysis of variance (time x groups) indicated a significant relationship of time. Mauchly's sphericity was significant at the $p<.05$ level therefore Huynh-Felt correction was utilized. $F(3.553,149.232)= 9.100$ $p<=.000$.

However, there was no significance between the type of treatment $F(3.553, 149.232) = .574$ $p = .661$. Results demonstrated that the use of both thermal ultrasound and shortwave diathermy produced a statistically significant effect on hamstring flexibility ROM over a period time.

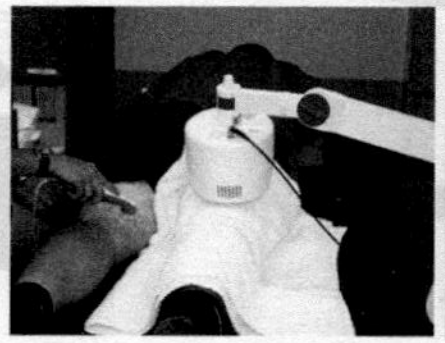

Figure 1. Therapeutic Modality Applications

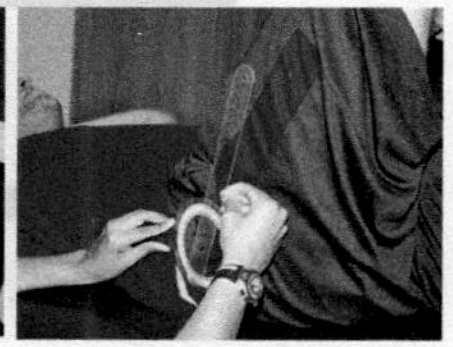

Figure 2. Hip Flexion ROM Evaluation

Tests of Within-Subjects Contrasts

Measure: ROM

Source	Time	Type III Sum of Squares	df	Mean Square	F	Sig.	Partial Eta Squared	Noncent. Parameter
Time	Linear	12.784	1	12.784	.869	.357	.020	.869
	Quadratic	310.015	1	310.015	23.966	.000	.363	23.966
	Cubic	58.182	1	58.182	5.347	.026	.113	5.347
	Order 4	14.047	1	14.047	2.880	.097	.064	2.880
Time * Group	Linear	9.020	1	9.020	.613	.438	.014	.613
	Quadratic	11.183	1	11.183	.865	.358	.020	.865
	Cubic	4.400	1	4.400	.404	.528	.010	.404
	Order 4	.332	1	.332	.068	.795	.002	.068
Error (Time)	Linear	618.095	42	14.717				
	Quadratic	543.302	42	12.936				
	Cubic	457.018	42	10.881				
	Order 4	204.821	42	4.877				

Discussion and Summary

Flexibility is important in prevention of sports injuries, as lack of it is a predisposing factor to musculoskeletal injuries. Athletes with increased tightness of the hamstring muscle group have a statistically higher risk for musculoskeletal lesions. The most widely used method to increase range of motion is stretching, but research has demonstrated that the use of thermal modalities can be implemented to increase flexibility and decrease joint stiffness. This research study was geared to inform clinicians of the most appropriate and effective ways to promote increases in flexibility, to then in turn, decrease the risk of injury. Interpretation of the data allowed the conclusion that neither thermal ultrasound or shortwave diathermy was more effective than the other. In this study, both modality choices demonstrated to be effective thermal modalities that increased hip flexion ROM significantly after the treatment concluded. Furthermore, the diathermy and the ultrasound modality should be considered appropriate treatments when a clinician is concerned with increasing a patient's flexibility.

The results of this study demonstrated that the use of both thermal ultrasound and shortwave diathermy produced a statistically significant effect on hamstring flexibility range of motion over a period time. Although range of motion increased, there was no significant difference between the increases in range of motion when comparing the two modalities; shortwave diathermy and thermal ultrasound. Regardless of which treatment intervention used, the results suggested that flexibility exercise should be initiated immediately up to 2 minutes following the modality treatment for maximal benefit. This is shown through the decreases in flexibility when measured five minutes post modality treatment.

References

1. Akbari A, Moodi H, Moein A, Nazok R. The effect of therapeutic ultrasound and duration of stretching of the hamstring muscle group on the passive knee extension. *J Med Sci.* 2006;6(6), 968-973.
2. Draper D, Castro J, Feland B, Schulthies S, Eggett D. Shortwave diathermy and prolonged stretching increase hamstring flexibility more than prolonged stretching alone. *J Orthop Sports Phys Ther.* 2004;34(1), 13-20.
3. Ahmed E, Alghamdy M, Almalky M. Comparative effect of the ultrasound therapy versus static stretching on the extensibility of hamstring muscles. *Int J Med Sci Public Health.* 2014;3(4), 466-471.
4. Draper D, Knight K, Fujiwara T, Castel C. Temperature change in human muscle during and after pulsed short-wave diathermy. *J Orthop Sports Phys Ther.* 1999;29(1):13-22
5. Draper D, Miner L, Knight K, Ricard M. The carry-over effects of diathermy and stretching in developing hamstring flexibility. *J Athl Train.* 2002;37(1), 37-42.
6. Brucker J, Knight K, Rubley M, Draper D. An 18-day stretching regimen, with or without pulsed, shortwave diathermy, and ankle dorsiflexion after 3 weeks. *J Athl Train.* 2005;40(4):276-280
7. Martinez-Rodriguez A, Bello O, Yanez-Brage I. Effect of a Single Pulsed Shortwave Diathermy Treatment on Extensibility of the Hamstrings. *Int J Athl Ther Train.* 2014;19(1):6-10
8. Gajdosik RL, Bohannon RW. Clinical measurement of range of motion. Review of goniometry emphasizing reliability and validity. *Phys Ther.* 1987; 67(12):1867-72
9. Konor MM, Morton S, Eckerson JM, Grindstaff TL. Reliability of three measures of ankle dorsiflexion range of motion. *Int J Sports Phys Ther.* 2012; 7(3):279-87

Poster 12-6. Text-heavy poster. (Reprinted with permission from Dr. Kelley Henderson, EdD, LAT, ATC.)

Sidebar 12-3

As the instructor of a writing-intensive course, students were required to construct and a present their culminating project at our university's undergraduate research symposium. One student had worked diligently on poster design and construction on her MAC and was ready to print. She did not take the time to print a sample on our department computer to ensure all spacing and colors were appearing as she desired. She sent the file to the print shop and was informed the next day that it was ready for pickup. She went to view it and realized that her text was running past the lower borders of the text boxes in several places, making it difficult to read, as well as throwing off the overall aesthetic appearance of the poster. She asked the printer why that may have happened, and only then did she realize that the print shop software was not fully compatible with MAC-constructed PowerPoint slides. For other projects, we now recommend that all posters be emailed to faculty for review of appearance prior to the print shop, as well as all must be printed in smaller scale at least 3 times to confirm accurate display of all content.

Transporting the Poster

Following printing, authors will need to transport the poster to the presentation. At all times, this should be in a protected case to avoid exposure to the elements as well as the possibility of general wear and tear. Rolling the poster should be done with care, ensuring the edges match. It may be beneficial to roll the poster print-side out so that the edges will lay flat against the display board rather than curl inward.

Presenting the Poster

After all of the hard work to construct the poster, authors will finally arrive at a point during which they can display and present their poster. Prior to arrival, authors should ensure that they have read the guidelines for when the poster is to be displayed, put the poster up on time, and remove the poster when instructed. Poster authors do not want to have theirs be the last poster left up at the end of a presentation period, hours after the window for display has expired and possibly preventing the author from retrieving his or her poster due to limited access to the poster area.

As stated in Sidebar 12-4, bring thumb tacks or other display-hanging materials as there is no guarantee that these items will be provided in ample supply to properly support the poster. Authors should consider their poster color scheme and select hanging materials that will compliment, rather than distract from, the overall aesthetic construction. Also, bring a friend! Rolling the poster out and tacking it onto the provided stand is much easier with 2 people. It may help to attach the top corners evenly first, smooth down the center of the poster, and then secure the bottom corners. Other tips of the poster design, construction, and presentation process are provided in Table 12-8.

Prior to presenting, practice describing the project and the poster in advance. Rehearse a few sentences that provide an overview of the project.[4] This preparation will allow authors to be more confident in discussion with those viewing the poster. Specifically, think ahead to the types of questions readers may ask, and consider preparing a few questions to ask those that view the poster, including asking for their input specific to findings and key points. The more comfortable an author is with his or her material (specifically, the limitations and discussion points), the more seamless the responses will be. Authors should be encouraging dialog and exchange with those that view the poster, including taking the opportunity to interact with the poster. For example, use of clear gestures or touching the results section could illustrate the findings more intently to the reader. Neither the author nor the reader should be afraid to touch the poster.

Sidebar 12-4

How to travel with a poster:

- Never fold the poster; instead, roll it print-side out, making sure all edges align.
- Secure the poster with a rubber band in the middle rather than paper clips at the edges.
- Obtain a tube that will allow for the rolled poster to fit well and be protected.
- If traveling by plane, carry the poster on; do not check it in case it gets lost, resulting in a missed opportunity to present.
- If traveling an extremely far distance or if there are many posters to transport, consider shipping the posters, with tracking numbers, in advance of the presentation.
- Pack thumb tacks in order to secure the poster on the board.

Table 12-8. Poster Consideration Top 10 List

RESEARCHER ADVICE: TOP 10 CONSIDERATIONS FOR POSTER CONSTRUCTION AND PRESENTATION	
10	Identify the target audience for the poster, and aim the product toward them.
9	Consistency is key—font size, header construction, punctuation, borders, etc.
8	Keep the title manageable—less than 16 words if possible; consider whether the answer to the research question should be "given away" in the title.
7	Ensure the purpose statement of the project is clearly identified and bolded.
6	Include a graphic and/or photo to catch the reader's attention; be sure it is relevant and enhances the quality of the poster.
5	Be sure the font is readable from at least 4 feet away—typically no smaller than 24-point font in PowerPoint
4	Keep interactions with the poster in mind; it is a poster, not a chandelier.
3	Spelling errors are unacceptable.
2	Print out a sample on a smaller sheet at least once, and check for errors; do not let the first analysis of the full poster be after it is printed.
1	No last minute printing! Know in advance where the poster will be printed and how much lead time is needed for printing.

In summary, the poster presents authors with an opportunity to tell the story of their work. Once the draft of the poster has been created, authors are encouraged to edit and revise it as needed—get others to view the poster and provide critiques prior to printing. Utilizing the guidelines outlined in this chapter should enhance the authors ability to share their information in a creative manner while highlighting important findings.

Acknowledgments

The author would like to thank Dr. Sarah E. Wallace and Dr. Erica Beidler for their insight during the development of this chapter.

References

1. Theuner G, Pischke K, Bley T. Analysis of advertising effectiveness with eye tracking. Proceedings of Measuring Behavior, 2008; August 26-29, 2008; Maastricht, The Netherlands. http://www.noldus.com/mb2008/individual_papers/FPS_eye_tracking/FPS_eye_tracking_Theuner.pdf

2. Hess G, Tosney K, Liegel L. *Creating Effective Poster Presentations: AMEE Guide No 40.* Dundee, UK: Association for Medical Education in Europe; 2009.

3. Beilenson J. Developing effective poster presentations. *Gerontology News.* 2004;32(9):6-9.

4. Miller JE. Special articles: capacity building for health services research: preparing and presenting effective research posters. *Health Res Educ Trust.* 2007;42(1):311-328.

5. Nelson DE, Brownson RC, Remington PL, Parvanta C, eds. *Communicating Public Health Information Effectively: A Guide for Practitioners.* Washington, DC: American Public Health Association; 2002.

6. American College of Sports Medicine. ACSM annual meeting: instructions for poster presentations and thematic poster presentations. http://www.acsmannualmeeting.org/wp-content/uploads/2015/12/2017-Poster-and-Thematic-Poster-Instructions.pdf. Accessed September 30, 2017.

7. National Athletic Trainers' Association, Research and Education Foundation. Free communications program guidelines and recommendations: poster presentations. https://natafoundation.org/wp-content/uploads/Poster_Guidelines.pdf. Accessed September 30, 2017.

8. Galfano G, Dalmaso M, Marzoli D, Pavan G, Coricelli C, Castelli L. Eye gaze cannot be ignored (but neither can arrows). *Q J Exp Psychol (Hove).* 2012;65(10):1895-1910.

9. Nielsen J. F-shaped pattern of reading web content. *Nielsen Norman Group.* https://www.nngroup.com/articles/f-shaped-pattern-reading-web-content-discovered. Published April 17, 2006.

10. Bejan A. The golden ratio predicted: vision, cognition and locomotion as a single design in nature. *Int J Des Nat Ecodyn.* 2009;4(2):97-104.

11. University of Liverpool. *Making an Impact With Your Poster.* Liverpool, UK: University of Liverpool, Computing Services; 2012.

12. Davis, M. *Scientific Papers and Presentations.* New York, NY: Academic Press; 1997.

13. Gosling PJ. *Scientist's Guide to Poster Presentation.* Berlin, Germany: Springer Science + Business Media, LLC; 1997.

14. Briscoe M. *Preparing Scientific Illustrations: A Guide to Better Posters, Presentations, and Publications.* 2nd ed. New York, NY: Springer; 1996.

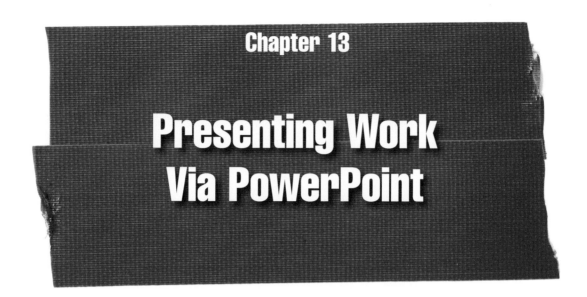

Chapter 13

Presenting Work Via PowerPoint

Jennifer M. Medina McKeon, PhD, ATC, CSCS

Similar to a poster presentation, an oral presentation—with accompanying slideshow—requires a different writing style than a research paper. This chapter will focus on how to transfer thoughts from a carefully worded paper onto a presentation medium and still retain the message. The chapter author will focus on guiding the reader on how to convert ideas into bullet points and still ensure proper flow as well as being able to extract the most relevant points from the original paper. Sports medicine and kinesiology-based examples and sample problems in this chapter will mimic Chapter 12 in that they will focus on creating an effective bullet point, understanding which concepts to take from a paper, and how and when to develop new material for a presentation to better set up the concept used from the original paper.

Good oral presentation involves a coordinated effort amongst the slides, practice, and delivery. All 3 should complement each other and not be seen independently. In the following sections, information on effective slide design, purposeful practice, and successful delivery will be discussed.

Designing the Slides

The first step for the presentation is designing the slides. This should go beyond just opening up presentation software and typing away. Thoughtful planning of the slideshow is a must in order to maximize the message delivery. Within this section, there are specific points and tips to consider in order to create the most effective presentation. Please note that Figures 13-1 and 13-2 are an example of a poorly designed slide and a fairly well-designed slide. There are many errors on the first that are corrected in the second slide. After reading this section, see how many can be identified.

Knoblauch M. *Professional Writing in
Kinesiology and Sports Medicine* (pp 149-174).
© 2019 Taylor & Francis Group.

Figure 13-1. Poorly designed slide.

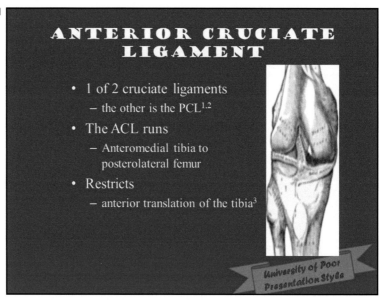

Figure 13-2. Fairly well-designed slide.

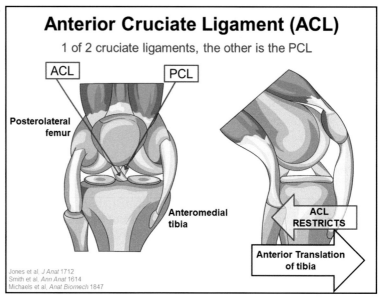

The Nuts and Bolts: Slide Number and Size

When creating a slideshow, there are a couple of preliminary steps even before visual design. These are the length of the presentation and size of the slides. Considering these 2 items first can potentially save a great deal of hassle down the road by ensuring that the designed slideshow actually matches with what is needed.

Do Not Exceed the Allotted Time

Mistakes in presentation are often the result of poor planning. Nothing reveals poor planning in a presentation as much as going over allotted time. It is important for presenters to know themselves—do they stick to the "script," do they like to improvise, do they speak slowly, do they rush when nervous? This is the first step to good planning.

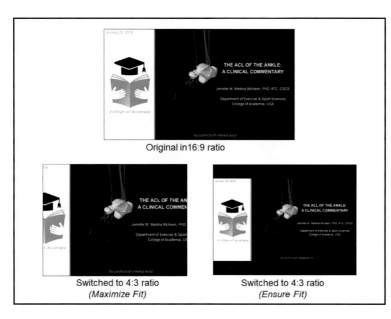

Figure 13-3. Original slide size, and then resized with maximize fit and ensure fit.

As a rule of thumb, keep the number of slides developed to about 67% to 75% of the allotted time. For example, if giving a 15-minute talk, there should be no more than about 12 slides total. For a 60-minute talk, no more than approximately 45 slides total. This includes the title slide and the thank you slide. If there will be slides with tables or figures, cut back even further as these take extra time to go through (see the Tables and Figures section in this chapter for further information). Are there videos? Again, be sure to leave some extra time (see the section on Videos). Are there builds (see the section on Builds)? Each build may account for another slide and must be included in the slide count as well.

It may feel as though there may not be enough things to say, but this will not happen. If anything goes wrong with the timing of the presentation, it will be that time seems to go too quickly, leaving the presenter to rush through the end of the presentation, right when the best material is coming up. Even if there is an extra moment or 2 at the end, this extra time can be used very effectively to conclude gracefully and answer questions (see the End It section toward the end of this chapter).

If the Slide Fits …

In the beginning of software-based presentation design, the slide size was fairly standard. A 4:3 width-to-height ratio was the default design. Therefore, there was little concern for slides to become jumbled when reformatted to a different slide size. Currently, there are additional and common default sizes. If slides are designed on one size setting and then opened on another, the visual material can become reformatted, and beautifully designed slides can look terrible. The "ensure fit" (or similar) function can help to make sure everything fits, but can sometimes also wreak havoc on the content design (Figure 13-3). One nearly surefire way to prevent visual reformatting is to contact the presentation organizers to see what slide size format will be used, and design the slides accordingly.

Slides Are Not Notecards

One of the worst things about many presentations is that the default design for presentations (a bulleted outline notecard) led to almost everyone treating that format as the default way to present information. This has led to years of boring, rote, uninteresting presentations that the audience members passively stare at (with a bit of drool coming out of their mouths) as they vaguely listen

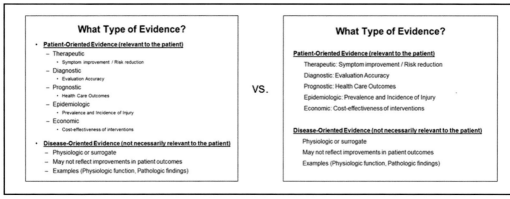

Figure 13-4. Unnecessary use of bullets and then a similar slide with bullets removed.

to a speaker drone on through the notecards that they have put up on the screen for everyone to see. Even worse, the poor presenter sometimes just reads the bullets, leading to a choppy, stilted performance. Even if a presenter feels that this presentation style describes him or her, it is essential to break this habit in any way possible.

Bullets are the worst! Rather, a bulleted *outline* presentation is the worst; slides are not note-cards! Presenters should understand that, despite the default design when opening up their presentation application (a rectangular placeholder with bulleted outline), this is a terrible use of the space available to assist in the message delivery. Bullets kill people and bulleted outlines kill presentations.

Bullets (Notes and Lists) Versus Statements (Sentences) Versus Messages (What Is Meant to Be Conveyed)

When designing slides, particular consideration for *what* and *why* elements will be included on a slide is crucial. First, consider the worded elements (visuals will come later). Scripted communication can be divided into lists, statements, and messages.

- For Lists: Bulleted or non-bulleted lists can be used sparingly and meaningfully. An example of a purposeful and appropriate use for bullets is if the presenter is creating a list. Even within these lists, an actual bullet is not always needed. See Figure 13-4 for an example of listing information without actually using bullets next to each statement.

- For Statements: Occasionally, a full statement is warranted; in other words, a complete or nearly complete sentence is needed. The rationale for using a full sentence is when an exact meaning or phrasing needs to be communicated to the audience. For example, using a specific, famous quote might be a time where a statement is necessary. If using a statement, it is a chance to slow down and read the *exact* statement, with emphasis on the key items to be highlighted. It may be preferable to change the font color or weight to correspond with points of emphasis, further assisting in tying visual performance to verbal performance. For example:

  Placebos can improve symptoms, which can be characterized as healing from a patient-centered perspective

  Placebos can improve symptoms, *which can be characterized as* healing *from a patient-centered perspective*

  From these examples, even in print, the emphasis in the second version can be felt. If read aloud with that same emphasis, the message will be strengthened for the audience.

- For Messages: The message should be first and foremost when slides are being developed. For each slide, questions related to "Is the message clear?" should be asked, such as "Is this truly the best way this message can be presented?" or "Is there a better, clearer, more concise manner in which this message can be communicated?" Apply the "packing a suitcase" strategy to each: can half be taken out and still be appropriate to compliment what is spoken verbally? At first, this can seem tedious, especially when applied to each slide. However, with an active approach to this process and a bit of practice, this will become second nature. When "recycling" an older lecture, take the time to go through it and look for slides that could be revised to more clearly present the necessary information.

Visuals

Amongst the most important elements to consider on slides are the visuals. *Visuals* go beyond just the images; the visuals are a way to think about how the entire canvas of a slide is arranged to maximize clarity of the message. Images should be included in this consideration, in conjunction with the placeholders, white space, background images, and builds.

Background Space: Placeholder and the "White Space"

The background is the entire space on the slide. This includes the *placeholder*, the box that holds the presenter's text, and the *white space*, the space around the text and images and elements. This space should be used appropriately. The default text box that pops up when opening a new slideshow document is actually very small compared to the entirety of the slide space. It wastes a great deal of space around the edges of the slide while simultaneously diminishing the amount of text space that is available. The result is a small, crammed text box that is floating mid-space in the slide. Consider expanding the size of a text box, providing more space, and also moving the text box to a better location on the slide. If feeling particularly creative, start with a completely blank slide and add text boxes where they are wanted and necessary.

Background Images and Removing Them

Background images are often included by default on slides that were designed by a media department for many institutions. In truth, these do look good and continually highlight the institution throughout the slideshow. However, there are times when the words within the text boxes or other images cut across that background image. This is visually displeasing. It is possible to turn off the background images on an individual slide when this happens. This looks better than partially covering the background images with text, images, or figures, or when using a different colored background. The background image will show up again on the subsequent slides if configured properly. See Figure 13-1 for overlapped background images.

Images

It is said that "a picture is worth 1000 words," and there certainly should not be 1000 words on a slide. Purposeful images should be used extensively, but judiciously. The images that are put on the slide should enhance the message, complement what is being said, and further explain a difficult concept. Random pictures of animals, the presenter's kids, or a favorite sports team are distracting and do not have a place within the main presentation. While this seems obvious, it is amazing how often this happens. The images should enhance, not detract from, the message.

Image Placement

Image placement on the slide is an important consideration. The default placeholder for an image is centrally to the left or to the right of the text (see Figures 13-1 and 13-5). It is an easy trap to click one of these default "image" slides and then to stick a picture in there that is peripherally related to the text or message, and then to repeat this, ad nauseum, through the end of the

Figure 13-5. Slide with image on top. This image has a border.

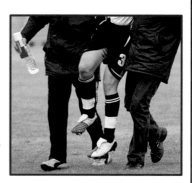

Figure 13-6. Slide with image as part of the background.

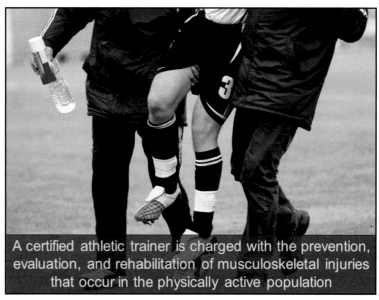

presentation. Consider moving the image by, for example, centering it on the slide and placing text around it.

Relative to the background, images can be placed *on* the background (see Figures 13-1 and 13-5), be *part of* the background (see Figure 13-2), or *be* the background itself (Figure 13-6). Images on the background tend to be the most common placement for images. This is the typical setup, when the image gets inserted into the placeholder. It is similar to gluing a picture onto a poster board collage—the picture is situated on top of the background. Images can become a part of the background when the background color and the image background color are the same (see Figure 13-2). The background surrounding the knee is white, matching the slide background. The result is the impression that the knee is at an equal visual level with the white slide background. However, if that same knee image, with the white background is placed on a blue background, the result is the impression that the image is on top, as previously described. Images with invisible backgrounds are particularly useful since they can be placed on any color background and still give the appearance of being a part of the slide. One consideration: be sure that the image's colors do not clash horribly with the background or become too distracting. If that is the case, change the background color, even if it just for that slide. Color will be addressed further in a following section. Finally, it can be visually appealing and impactful to make the image into the background itself (see Figure 13-6).

Image Borders

When an image is inserted into a slide, it typically does not have a border around it. Putting a line or border around the image will sharpen up the way that the slide looks (see Figures 13-1 [no border] vs 13-5 [with border]). The border line does not need to be decorative (fancy) or very wide, but a simple line can improve the overall finished look to the slide.

Image Size and Proportionality

Two important considerations are image size (the number of pixels) and image proportionality. The size of the image is relevant, especially when the image projected on the big screen will be much larger than when on the computer screen. An image that is too small—too few pixels, not overall length and height—will appear blurry or "pixelated." If using images taken with a camera or phone, be sure that each has selected to capture the image in a high resolution to avoid pixelating the image. If using images from the internet, be sure to search images that are labeled as "large" or "extra large." On most search engines, there is a way to select the size of the image needed. The image size is presented as the image dimensions (eg, 960 × 720). By opening the "Properties" menu for an image file, the presenter can check the image dimensions. Images with dimensions over 720 × 720 pixels generally show well for presentations. While these increase the overall file size of the slide show, it is well worth the extra bytes of memory.

Similarly, if an image to be used does not fit on the slide exactly as needed, be sure to reduce or expand the size proportionally (ie, maintain "aspect ratio"). An image that is stretched or squeezed in one direction (lengthwise or widthwise) and not proportionally looks unprofessional. Another option for pictures that do not fit as needed is to crop the image to the size that is needed, ensuring that important information is not cropped out. See Figures 13-1 and 13-2 for correct vs incorrect consideration for image pixel size and proportion.

Tables and Figures

As a general rule, use a figure whenever possible. Graphs, charts, and images are much more easily understood by the audience than words or numbers. Tables with "real numbers" in them can be very hard to interpret meaning in a presentation format and, as such, should be used sparingly. Further, if a table absolutely must be used, keep the number of significant digits under control. Is there really a difference between 0.7 and 0.7342? If not, then do not report it as such; too many decimal places just adds clutter, making the message more unclear (Figure 13-7). Be sure to clearly label all elements on all tables or figures to clarify their meaning. Figures 13-8 vs 13-9 and Figures 13-10 vs 13-11 are examples.

Fonts

Font selection can be as important as the words that are written in that font. Fonts that are distracting, difficult to read, or childish-appearing (if that is not the goal), detract from the intended message. For the following, it will be assumed that the goal is to develop a professional presentation, and for that, only a professional font will be appropriate.

Figure 13-7. Too much data in a table vs using figures to describe results.

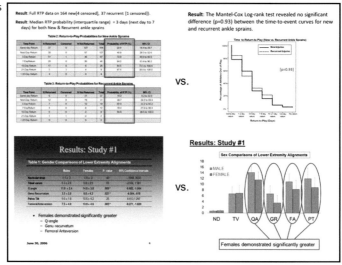

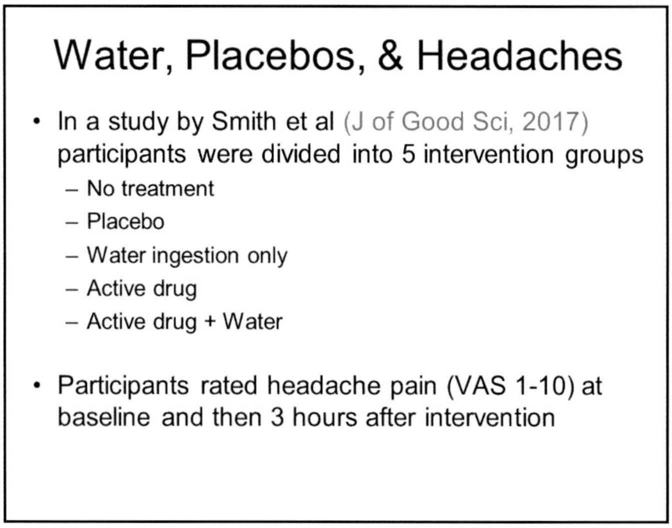

Figure 13-8. An example of a poor use of bullets and numbers to describe experimental design with results.

Water, Placebos, & Headaches

- In a study by Smith et al (J of Good Sci, 2017) participants were divided into 5 intervention groups
  - No treatment
  - Placebo
  - Water ingestion only
  - Active drug
  - Active drug + Water

- Participants rated headache pain (VAS 1-10) at baseline and then 3 hours after intervention

Figure 13-9. An example of a better use of experimental design with results as a graphic.

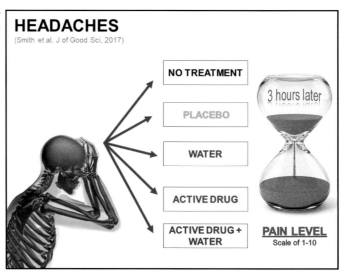

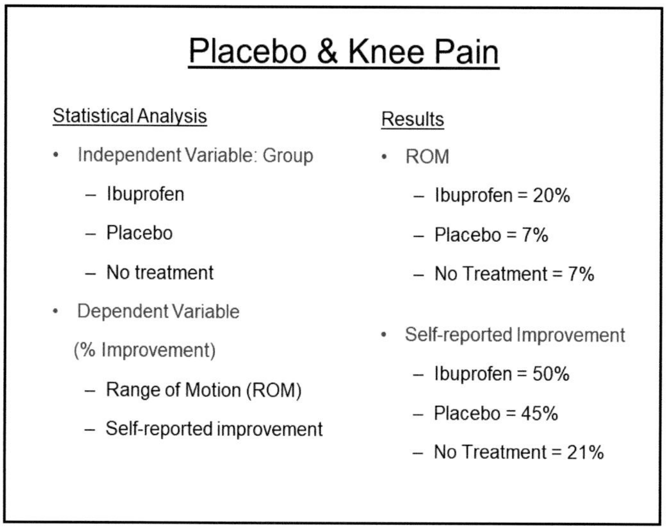

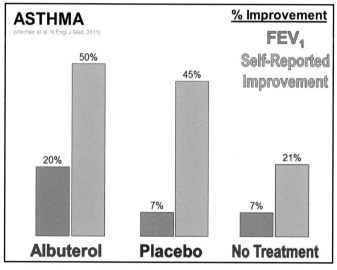

Placebo & Knee Pain

Statistical Analysis

- Independent Variable: Group
  - Ibuprofen
  - Placebo
  - No treatment
- Dependent Variable
  (% Improvement)
  - Range of Motion (ROM)
  - Self-reported improvement

Results

- ROM
  - Ibuprofen = 20%
  - Placebo = 7%
  - No Treatment = 7%
- Self-reported Improvement
  - Ibuprofen = 50%
  - Placebo = 45%
  - No Treatment = 21%

Figure 13-10. A second example of poor use of bullets and numbers to describe experimental design with results.

ASTHMA
(Wechler et al, N Engl J Med, 2011)

% Improvement

FEV_1

Self-Reported Improvement

50%

45%

20%

7%

7%

21%

Albuterol   **Placebo**   **No Treatment**

Figure 13-11. A second example of a better use of experimental design with results as a graphic.

Serifs Versus Sans Serifs: What Is a "Serif" and Why Does That Matter?

Once the difficult-to-read, distracting, and childish fonts are eliminated as options, there are still several professional-looking options available. These can be broadly classified into *serif* and *sans serif* fonts. Simply, "serifs" are the little feet that are at the base of the letters for some fonts (Figure 13-12). Probably the most familiar serif font is Times New Roman. In addition to the "feet," the line weight (thickness) of an individual letter varies, with some parts of a letter being thicker than others. A sans serif font lacks these feet and also has a consistent line weight throughout the letter. A commonly known sans serif font is Arial. While both are often used in presentations, sans serif fonts tend to be easier to read on a presentation. Part of this has to do with how the narrower line weights bleed and blend into the background, leaving almost "gaps" in the letters. Not to totally disparage serif fonts, they are actually very good selections when reading long sections of written text, such as in a book or many journal articles. See Figures 13-1 vs 13-2 for the contrast between serif and sans serif fonts.

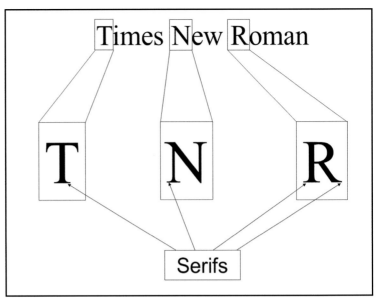

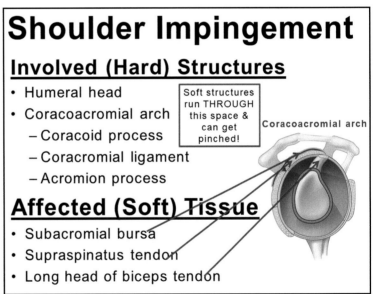

Font Size—People Have to Be Able to Read It

Font size is an important consideration and, interestingly, both too small and too big can be difficult to read. Too small is obvious; people have to squint to see it, and small font can be problematic to the individuals in the back of the room. In contrast, too big or too spread out is also hard to read; it is difficult for the brain to recognize the familiar patterns that it is used to when reading (Figure 13-13).

Increasing the font size can help to emphasize a point or be used to create a header. Decreasing the font size might be used to make a small side note or indicate a referenced citation. For font size changes within a slide, the Rule of 3 applies here—generally, no more than 3 different font sizes per slide (Sidebar 13-1). Further, if changing font sizes, it is generally good practice to give at least an 8-point difference between sizes. This will make the font size change appear intentional; less than an 8-point change is noticeable but can look like it was a formatting mistake.

Sidebar 13-1

Rule of 3

One concept to remember for font size selection, color, and levels of bulleted outline is the Rule of 3. No more than 3 different font sizes, no more than 3 colors, and no more than 3 levels of bulleted outline should be used per slide.

References

One consideration is referencing within a slideshow. In many research presentations, it is appropriate and necessary. However, the way that referencing is done can change the impact of those references. For the sake of space, many times, referencing is accomplished in a manner similar to a journal article: a superscripted number at the end of the statement (see Figure 13-1), with a reference "section" (slide) at the end of the presentation. Unfortunately, that reference slide gets flipped through very quickly ("These are my references, any questions?") and provide no valuable information to the audience. A preferable approach is to insert basic citation information directly onto the respective slide (see Figure 13-2). This way, the listener can connect the citation directly to the information presented.

Spellcheck the Slides

Although not directly related to the font, it would be remiss to not mention spellchecking the slides. Review each slide carefully for inaccuracies, poor grammar, and incorrect spelling—this one is self-explanatory! After several reviews, a certain level of fatigue sets in and errors might be missed. Get a friend or colleague to take a look if it seems that review fatigue is setting in. When a spelling error is seen in 9-inch tall letters, it can be very distracting. It can also call into question the credibility of the presenter or the care with which the presenter prepared for the talk.

Colors

Color selection is important to consider throughout the slide design process. The science of color is actually very interesting, and a few basic pieces of information can help with color selection for the slide. For color, the terms *hue*, *tint*, *shade*, and *tone* are ones that have specific meanings to them. Hue essentially means "color." Red, blue, etc are all hues. A simple color wheel (Figure 13-14) illustrates the primary and secondary colors. Primary colors are red, blue, and yellow. Secondary colors, orange, purple, and green, are the 3 colors formed by mixing 2 of the primary colors. Selective combinations of certain colors can help with delivering the wanted message. Tints and shades are when white or black, respectively, is added to the hue (see Figure 13-14). Tones are essentially adding gray (both black and white) to a color, in varying amounts of black or white. Four other concepts can assist with color selection: achromatic, monochromatic, analogous, and complementary. For achromatic slides (Figure 13-15), no hues are used, just various degrees of black and white. For monochromatic slides, one hue (color) is used with varying degrees of tint and shade to that hue (Figure 13-16). For slides using an analogous scheme, 2 to 3 hues that are adjacent on the color wheel are used (Figure 13-17). Slides with a complementary color scheme use 2 colors that are on the opposite sides of the color wheel (Figure 13-17). Any of these 4 styles can be effective and visually appealing; overdoing it or combining schemes can be overwhelming. In any case, the Rule of 3 applies here, again—no more than 3 colors per slide. Lastly, remember the Hippocratic Oath of Color: If color cannot be used wisely, it is best to avoid it entirely. Above all, do no harm (Figure 13-18).

Figure 13-14. The color wheel, with primary and secondary colors. Following, the color wheel in shades and tints.

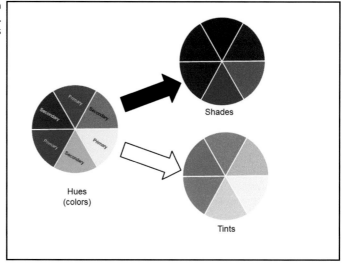

Figure 13-15. An example of an achromatic color scheme.

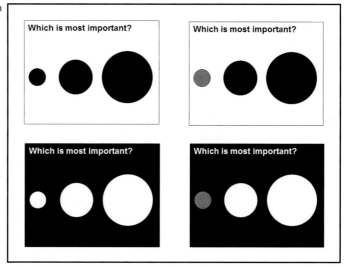

Figure 13-16. An example of a monochromatic color scheme.

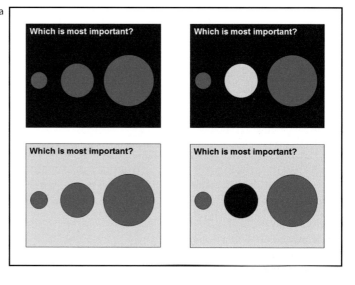

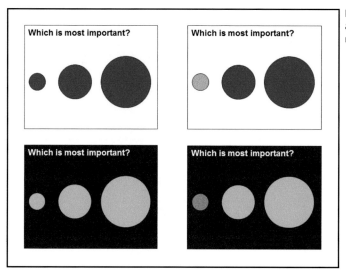

Figure 13-17. An example of an analogous color scheme and complementary color scheme.

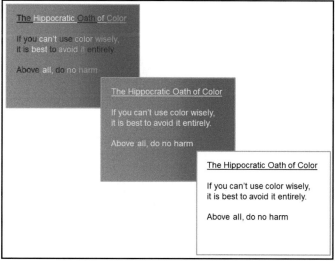

Figure 13-18. The Hippocratic Oath of Color.

Background Versus Font

Black and white are obviously the most contrasting colors that can be used on a slide. White font on a black background, or vice versa, shows very well. In general, colors that have very different value (the lightness or darkness of the colors) will be easier to see (eg, light-colored font on a dark background or dark-colored fonts on a light background are common selections). One key exception, is red. Red is a funny color; it is very conspicuous. It stands out and is easily seen; fire engines and stop signs are red for a reason. However, on a slideshow, red fonts and backgrounds should be used with caution. A red background can be overwhelming to the audience, induce eye strain, and even, as some research indicates, incite anger or aggressiveness. On a white background, or sometimes on black, red font can work. However, on a color background, red font is very difficult to read; the letters almost seem to squiggle and move on the slide. Besides red, there are definite color combinations that may or may not work. Test out a few to see what works best. In general, many audiences prefer darker backgrounds, but this may limit how images might show or how many colored fonts can be used. In any case, choose a background color with intention. The background and font colors should contrast well so that the words are not lost in the background. Figures 13-19 vs 13-20 are examples of poor vs reasonable color selection.

Figure 13-19. Examples of poor background and font color selections.

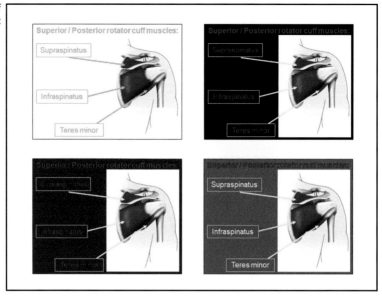

Figure 13-20. Examples of better choices of background and font color.

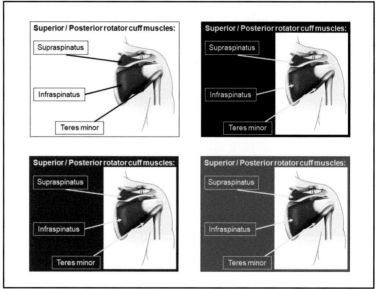

Complementing, Rather Than Competing With, the Message

Any visual used, whether image or words, should complement the message spoken by the presenter. Conflicting (or even off-topic) messages cause confusion; while the listeners are trying to figure out how the visual ties into the words spoken, they will be distracted (Figure 13-21). Further, the written words and images used should also be accompaniments for each other—not completely redundant, but sharing the workload of delivering the message.

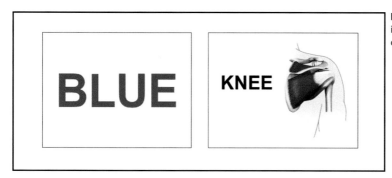

Figure 13-21. Conflicting information can lead to confusion.

Remember When …

Particularly for a longer presentation, it may be necessary for the audience to recall a previous piece of information, point, or theme. One way to facilitate this is to manipulate the background color to coordinate with specific themes. For example, if planning to present 2 to 3 individual case studies throughout a presentation, make the background color for those cases a different color. This will break up the monotony of the color scheme and also cue the audience into linking seemingly disparate information.

Builds

Builds are used to present smaller pieces of information sequentially rather than too much information all at once. The simplest example of this, within a slideshow, is to have individual bullets reveal themselves on a click. However, since bullet points are the worst, simply using them to reveal each point over and over on each identically designed slide will start to lose its impact. These builds should be just this, concentrated chunks of information that build into a larger or broader concept (Figure 13-22). Be sure to count each build as a separate slide (if necessary) so as to not go over the time limit.

Videos

Videos can be a great way to concisely explain certain difficult concepts, especially when describing body motion, task, or technique. However, there are some key things to remember when deciding to include a video.

Is a Video Absolutely Necessary?

While videos can help to explain certain information that is more visual in nature, they do take time to load up, play (a couple of times, because it almost always needs to be repeated to ensure that the audience caught all of the key elements), and also, explain. It seems that this can be done quickly, but usually takes longer than expected. For a short talk (eg, a 15-minute free communication), this can eat up a precious minute or 2.

Where Is the Video File?

The presenter should ensure that the file is included in the folder that holds the presentation or is directly embedded into the presentation. A video file that is in a different folder may not be "found" by the presentation file, and will not play. A good strategy is to put the presentation and the video file on a separate thumb drive, and then to try everything out on a different computer. See if everything will work when on a new computer at the podium. One consideration on directly embedding the videos: directly embedding the files can create an extremely large file size and might impede the ability for the presenter to self-email the file.

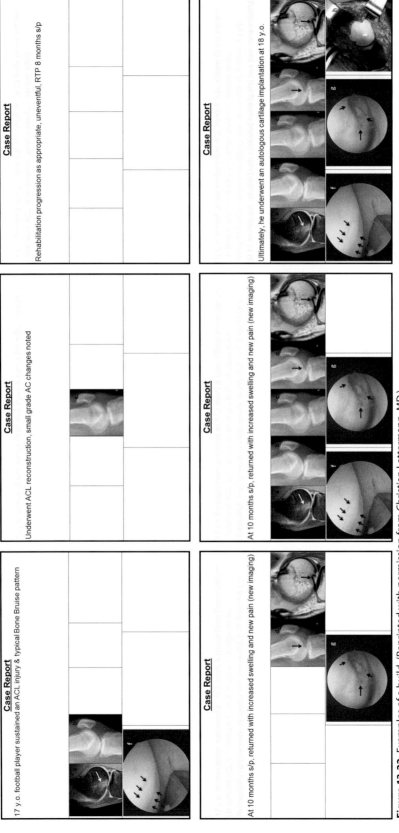

Case Report

17 y. o. football player sustained an ACL injury & typical Bone Bruise pattern

Case Report

Underwent ACL reconstruction, small grade AC changes noted

Case Report

Rehabilitation progression as appropriate, uneventful, RTP 8 months s/p

Case Report

At 10 months s/p, returned with increased swelling and new pain (new imaging)

Case Report

At 10 months s/p, returned with increased swelling and new pain (new imaging)

Case Report

Ultimately, he underwent an autologous cartilage implantation at 18 y.o.

Figure 13-22. Examples of a build. (Reprinted with permission from Christian Lattermann, MD.)

Who Is Going to "Play" the Video?

This leads to the next point: who plays the video is important to know. Be sure to take the time to check in with the IT personnel prior to the presentation time. Will presenters have access to play the video from the podium? Will they have to signal the IT member to play when needed? Will the thumb drive be used during the presentation or will it be uploaded from an offsite computer, along with having to upload the video, as well? Be sure to check on all of these items before going up to begin the presentation.

Is There Internet Access?

Similar to ensuring that a video file is located in the same file directory as the presentation, at times, an internet link may be embedded into the presentation to play an online video. Again, it is very important to check that that there will be reliable internet access during the presentation. If using one's own laptop, be sure that any access codes or passwords have been validated. Remember, linking over to the internet can take time; be sure as a presenter that this will not cost more minutes than needed.

What if the Video Does Not Play?

Ultimately, this is the question that the presenter must answer before deciding to include videos. If the presenter is new or somewhat uncomfortable with podium lectures, then the decision to include a video—which could easily go wrong—should be weighed carefully. If the presenter is okay with a video mishap, and that video is absolutely necessary, then go with it!

It seems that with everything that could go wrong, including videos may be a bad bet. In many cases, this is probably true. Be absolutely sure that a video is needed before including. However, when used appropriately, sparingly, and under the right conditions, videos can enhance a presentation substantially.

Perfecting the Delivery

Once the perfect slideshow is developed, the second, equally important task is to perfect the delivery. A visually pleasing slideshow, met with a classy, comfortable delivery results in a great presentation. Therefore, practicing that delivery—and practicing the correct way—is key to that great delivery.

Practice

A key point to practicing: there should be an inverse relationship to the time allotted compared to the time spent practicing. If the presenter has a couple of hours to speak, he or she can probably practice a bit less as there will be plenty of time to "correct" any missteps. However, with a short time allotment, the delivery has to be spot on; presenters get one chance to get their message right.

As an overview, practicing a presentation should include (minimally) these 3 steps:

1. Stand up: The presenter should find a place where he or she does not feel self-conscious. Put the slideshow on in presentation mode, and mark the time at which the presentation starts.
2. Say the words: Out loud, run through the presentation, just as if standing at a podium. Speak the words. Find out where stumbles may occur (I point out several common mistakes next; keep them in mind when doing these rehearsals). For the first time through, try not to start over. If there is a trip up or stumble or something that is not preferred on a slide, make a quick note and move on. These issues can be fixed prior to the next rehearsals.
3. Think like a lawyer: While reviewing slides, be sure that arguments and statements are sound. Be accurate within the information presented. Build a case, and support it throughout the

presentation (refer back to Chapter 1 on the art of rhetoric and developing good arguments). Think about the questions that audience members might ask. Would it be accepted as a reasonable answer? Would it be rejected as a superficial response? Inaccuracies or overgeneralizations are easily picked up by the audience and weaken arguments. If asked a question, give the complete answer, and get comfortable with saying "I don't know," which can always be followed up with " … but here is my best guess."

Tips for Practicing and Avoiding Common Mistakes When Preparing

Good practice includes doing the right things in a conscientious manner, not just going through the motions. In the following, there are several common mistakes that individuals make when preparing for a presentation. Now that so much time has been dedicated to developing visually appealing slides, it is time to commit a similar level of dedication to perfecting the delivery and avoiding these errors.

Exceeding the Allotted Time

While practicing, keep track of the time it takes to go through the talk. If a presenter keeps going over (or even cutting it really close) the time limit while practicing, he or she will likely go over or feel rushed at the end. When actually "live," there are time-eaters that are often forgotten about—conference proceedings running over time, the audience is not seated right when the talk is slotted to begin, moderators with lengthy introductions, etc. Practicing one's talk so that it is short by about 1 to 3 minutes (depending on the total time allotted) will ensure that it will adhere to the schedule. If a presenter does end up ahead by 1 minute or so, he or she should use that time to answer questions, expand on some key idea, or even, just end the presentation. Going under by 1 minute tends to go unnoticed. Going over, even by 1 minute, leads to uncomfortable shifting and gesturing by the moderator, and tends to garner wrath from the attendees and especially the next speaker.

"I Know What's on My Slides": The "Flip-Through" Method

"Oh, on this slide, umm … " One of the "flip-through" mistakes can occur when the speaker flips through slides that were created, focusing mainly on the words. An audience member can pick this one out easily. If anything has been learned up to this point, there should be far fewer words on the slide than those spoken to the audience. Reading only the words on the slide often leads to a stilted, somewhat incoherent message—there are too many gaps that are not being filled in with spoken words. The audience will also feel that this is a waste of time; they can read the slides as well as the presenter can. This is more often the mistake of someone more unfamiliar to public speaking. Be sure that the message comes through, not just words.

"I Don't Know What's on My Slides": The Other "Flip-Through" Method

Another, and sometimes more damning practice style, is the the speaker who "knows" what is on his or her slides and, therefore, never rehearses the actual words he or she needs to say. Overconfidence in the message but no practice in delivering that message can lead to stammering, repeating phrases, lots of distracting umms, and, generally, an incoherent message. In other words, there is an unpolished and unprepared result (Sidebar 13-2). The flip side of the previous point: practice the words, and beware of just memorizing the content and message.

According to Szewczyk et al …

Two errors that we tend not to think about in written manuscripts have to do with references. In written manuscripts, we can refer to an author as "Jones et al … " and move on from there without thinking too much about how to pronounce that name. If carelessly placed in a presentation, the

Sidebar 13-2

Practicing the Wrong Way!

I once witnessed this with disastrous results. I had picked up on the speaker's lack of preparation within 30 seconds or so: plenty of confidence at the start, and then the quick recognition that he could not go "off the cuff." However, (unpracticed) words failed the speaker and he panicked. An onstage meltdown proceeded, with the speaker cursing several times and then yelling at a colleague in the audience (during the talk). It was horrifically bad. I truly believe that the speaker knew the information through and through. In an informal setting, that individual could have probably pulled off a brilliant conversation about his given topic. However, on the spot, at the podium, without the casual give-and-take that occurs in a 2-way discussion, this speaker was stumped.

Sidebar 13-3

Pronunciation

I lived in Kentucky for a good while; however, I grew up far from that region of the country. While not the name of an individual (as far as I know), this is a story of getting a "common" name wrong. There are 2 towns in Kentucky, each with the spelling of famous cities across the Atlantic Ocean. The pronunciation is considerably different, however, and locals will (understandably) take exception to mispronunciation of Versailles [pronounced "Ver-sāyls"] and Athens [pronounced "Ā-thens"]. A mild embarrassment at the gas station when asking for directions could be amplified considerably if done in front of an audience of colleagues.

speaker may stumble upon an "unpronounceable" name, or worse, an uncommon pronunciation for a name that appears fairly common (Sidebar 13-3). Along that same line, the speaker should be able to correctly pronounce all words in the presentation.

A second error, is to assume that all cited authors are male. Of course, we know that is not true. However, in a presentation, when referring to a cited author, it may be easy to fall back into the male default. For example:

"Jones and colleagues did this really cool thing. Based on the results of his study … "

If Jones is male, that statement is fine. If Jones is female, that is a big and obvious mistake to many individuals in the audience. The presenter's credibility is in jeopardy. In research, it is common to search, cite, and discuss investigators by their last names only. Be sure to take a step back and ensure who each cited author is and how to pronounce all names before getting up on stage.

Getting Off to a Good Start

When practicing, be sure to not overlook the part of the talk that will set the tone for the rest of the time in front of the audience: getting off the title slide. Many speakers forget to practice this part and start off awkward and appearing unsure of what to say next. Why put oneself in a hole at the start? The audience appreciates the speaker who can come off as comfortable and humbly charismatic. See Sidebar 13-4 for some key steps to getting off on the right foot.

Working Through the Transitions Between Slides/Topics

Even with a full understanding of the slide content, one tricky area is transitioning from slide to slide. It is an easy trap—the key information on the slide is the most important part, but without smooth transitions, the presentation will appear stilted and not cohesive. Consider what will be

Sidebar 13-4

Options for Starting

Thank the moderator and the audience. Saying "thank you" is a great way to insert yourself into the presentation. Whoever introduces the presenter will finish. At that point, a quick thank you transfers the focus from the moderator, or emcee, to you in a smooth and polite manner. Optionally, you can next thank the audience. This is a nice gesture and can be done fairly quickly. I have included some options below that can easily be altered to fit any given circumstance.

For a regular presentation:

"Thank you for attending today … "

For an early morning presentation:

"Thank you for getting up early to attend … "

For a late day presentation:

"Thank you for sticking around … "

Thank your co-authors. If you have co-authors, you should thank them publicly. This includes inserting your co-author names on the title slide and then thanking them at the start of your talk. Here are a couple of options:

If you only have 1 or 2 co-authors:

"I'd like to thank my co-authors, John Smith and Mary Jones, for their contributions to this work (research, etc) … "

If you have several co-authors, you can forego naming them individually:

"I'd like to thank my co-authors for their contributions to this work (research, etc) … "

Introduce your topic/talk. It is okay to state your title, but you will need to have a couple of options. If the moderator steals your thunder and announces your title, you can still shift into introducing your topic in a clean way:

After thank you:

"Today, I'll be presenting on the evidence surrounding The Placebo Effect."

(If the moderator steals your opener):

Moderator: " … who will be presenting The Placebo Effect."

You: "Thank you, Jim. Today, I will be presenting on the biopsychosocial manifestations and clinical utility of understanding how placebos affect patients … "

Memorize these first few lines. Although it seems intuitive, be sure to have these title slide lines prepared and memorized. This will clear away any potential awkwardness and set you up for a smooth transition into what you know—your content.

said in-between slides to keep the flow of the presentation going. If, even with practice, there is not a clear transition from one slide to the next, then there is likely a piece missing in the story that is being told, and a modification to the presentation must be made to fill that gap.

End It

Have a graceful exit strategy. Prepare a clear conclusion to the presentation, succinctly summarizing major themes' key takeaway points. A rambling summary of the presentation or trailing off into a "well, that's the end" will be a letdown, even after a great presentation. A good touch is to have a final slide with contact information, allowing audience members to get in touch with the speaker if there are follow-up questions. Once finished, say thank you again, clearly and confidently. Following that, if there is time allotted, ask for questions.

Delivery

Now that the slides are developed and the presentation practiced, there are the on-site considerations. Within this section, there are steps and factors to think about to make a good impression while in front of the audience. These factors have to do with looking the part, sounding professional, and ensuring a comfortable presence at the podium.

Look Good

Most individuals know that they should "look good" or "dress professionally" while presenting, but what does that mean exactly? There are several pieces to consider—some, such as what to wear, need some preparation before arriving at the speaking engagement. Others should be in the back of the speaker's head throughout the talk. The more comfortable and prepared the speaker is with these elements, the more they will be second nature during the presentation.

Look the Part

Dressing up for a scientific presentation conveys 2 important messages. First, it conveys respect for those in the audience and the profession being represented. Second, it also signals a willingness to conform to standards set by the organization that invited the presenter to speak. The first—demonstrating respect for the audience and profession—is common sense. The audience will be more engaged in the material and forgiving across the performance if they believe that the speaker is respectful of their intellect and time. The second—conforming to protocol and standards—is not inherently bad. These boundaries exist for a reason, and staying within these confines is another method of tacitly conveying respect for the audience and the organization for which the presentation is being given.

Get Adjusted

The speaker should be positioned appropriately behind the microphone. Take a couple of moments to get comfortable behind the podium. Adjust the microphone so that it is at a comfortable height. If the microphone is too far or low, vocalizations will not be picked up consistently. If positioned too closely, certain consonant sounds (especially P and B) make a terrible "burst" sound against the microphone.

Stand Still

Nobody needs to be a statue behind the microphone. However, there are some movements that should be minimized. Swaying is one that many do when speaking to an audience. If distractive swaying is a problem, try standing in a stride stance (one foot in front of the other) behind the podium. This stance makes it difficult to sway and the presenter will stand still.

Along this line, if given more free range, the speaker should be aware of how much, how fast, and how far they tend to travel. A bit of motion is fine; pacing back and forth can be off-putting. Stopping for a moment, and standing still, can help to emphasize an important point.

Much of the preceding points will be directly affected by the type of microphone that is available. A podium microphone will tend to keep the speaker in the same place but may lend to swaying back and forth. A lapel microphone allows for more freedom but might encourage the speaker to pace unrestrictedly. Be aware of the pros and cons of each, and be prepared for either case.

Sound Good

Few people like the sound of their own voice when they hear it over the microphone. This can be somewhat surprising the first time when heard. Practicing the following will help the speaker develop a calm and confident speaker voice. Even without prior access to a microphone and audience, by becoming comfortable with a public speaking persona, the presenter will have more confidence when hearing his or her own voice booming over the loudspeakers.

Speak Up

The speaking volume should be slightly louder than conversational. Not shouting, of course, but it should be at a level that would feel uncomfortably loud if sitting right next to a person.

Think about projecting to the entire room rather than to the attendees in the front row only. Further, speak with controlled enthusiasm. The speaker should sound interested in the content of the talk. If the speaker sounds bored or boring, then the audience will be bored as well—guaranteed. Emphasizing key points and sounding sincerely interested will help to convince the audience that something important is being said. While there is some conflicting evidence regading the extent of the influence, research on the nonverbal characteristics that influence beliefs on speaker credibility and trustworthiness trace back almost a century. Among these nonverbal characteristics are varied intonation and inflection, which can be integrated into speech patterns. If unsure about how to practice varied intonation, think of an actor trying out various line readings:

"**Read** *that book*"

"*Read* **that** *book*"

"*Read that* **book**"

Notice the varying emphasis and how that changes the meaning of the statement. This is not to say that every line should be tested out as in the above example, but this is how the speaker can begin to consider how to emphasize, pause, and vary the manner of speaking.

Do Not Upspeak

Beware of this speech pattern. Many people (especially when nervous) will phrase every declarative sentence as a question. One sentence, spoken in this manner, can be overlooked. When up-speak is used continually, it gives the appearance that the speaker is unsure or unintelligent. Practice making statements as statements, not questions.

Use Appropriate Grammar When Speaking and on the Slides

This seems like common sense, but appropriate grammar on the slides (even for non-complete sentences) helps to create a polished and authoritative look and feel. Take the time to look for grammatical errors, colloquialisms, e-shorthand (the abbreviations that one often sees in popular social media), and other types of unprofessional speech or writing. The same is true for the words that are spoken. When speaking during the presentation, be aware of word use. Coming across as too casual will be a detriment to the credibility of the speaker.

Sidebar 13-5

Well, I Can See the Back of Your Head …

I once attended a presentation on the history of protective equipment in sport. The speaker even brought props—examples of older models of certain equipment. However, following the moderator's introduction, the speaker immediately turned his back on the audience and spoke directly to the projection screen for the entire lecture. Even when holding props and "demonstrating" and "pointing out" certain features, he did not turn around, and gestured to these features while obstructing the audience the entire time. Yikes!

Speak to the Audience

The speaker should be sure to speak to the audience. Good eye contact with audience members can be seen as an indicator of speaker credibility and trustworthiness. The presenter should actively seek out individuals and make direct eye contact and pause comfortably for a moment before searching for another individual. The speaker should avoid speaking directly to the computer or staring up at the projection screen. A glance at the monitor or display is fine, especially if describing a figure or image; however, the screen should not be the primary audience member. Along this same line, directly address individuals when answering questions—again, avoid looking at the display or the monitor during a question-or-answer period (Sidebar 13-5).

Identify With the Audience

In addition to speaking directly to the audience, the speaker should also identify with attendees. Think of the presentation as a dialogue with the audience, not just a monologue. Depending on the type of presentation, it can be good practice to stop and briefly engage with the audience directly, at times. Sometimes this might just be a call for questions or a query about whether something made sense. Again, depending on the type of presentation and topic, the speaker might want to ask of the attendees' own experiences with a given topic. If this tactic is employed, be prepared and consider the following during preparations:

- Be sure to incorporate this type of back-and-forth into timing during practice.
- Carefully plan how queries will be phrased to the audience; the presenter wants to be sure that the answers/comments that were being sought are the ones that come up.
- What is the contingency plan if no one answers? What will be the plan if someone goes on too long or if too many people want to comment?

On another note, many bigger conferences have rooms with dual presentations screens, one on each side of the speaker. Be sure not to lock into only one screen, especially with the pointer or when gesturing. This could potentially leave out half of the audience.

Slow and Steady … But Not Too Slow

With appropriate planning and practice, speaking should be even and measured—not boring, but comfortable. Speak at a comfortable pace. The presenter's posture at the podium should be composed and relaxed, not fidgety. Review the following points to ensure a strong presence during the presentation.

A Guiding Hand

Gesturing can add personality and emphasis, which are necessary to good presentation. Further, appropriate gestures may increase the audience's perception of the speaker's credibility. However, similar to excessive swaying or pacing, wild hand gesturing can be distracting to the audience. Further, overemphasizing with arm gestures can lead the speaker to accidentally strike

Sidebar 13-6

Slow, Slower, Slowest

For tables and figures, take an almost absurdly slow pace when explaining them. Here is a good rule of thumb: I once asked a friend how slow I should walk down the aisle as a bridesmaid at a wedding. Having more experience than me at that time, she replied, "Walk as slow as you can until it begins to feel silly. That is the right pace." To me, that is the way that tables and figures should be described while giving a presentation. Be sure to allot time for that while preparing.

the microphone and that terrible "burst" sound to be unleashed on the audience. An easy solution to this is for the speaker to put one hand in a coat or trousers/skirt pocket. With one hand in the pocket and the other holding a pointer, untoward gesturing might be kept to a minimum.

Laser Pointer Use

If available, use a laser pointer or mouse to make an indication toward important elements of the presentation. If unsure about whether one will be available, it makes sense to purchase and have one ready to go. While pointers are very useful, there are some items to consider:

- Hold the pointer with a steady hand and under control. If nervous and a bit shaky, audience members can see that with laser pointer use. An easy fix for that is to tuck the laser arm tight in against the body, and then flex the elbow and cross it across the body (almost like folding one's arms). This will stabilize the laser when using it.
- Use the pointer sparingly. Another trap that many speakers fall into is to point at every slide, every point. Usually, this is accompanied by a "swirl," another irritating motion when used repeatedly. Sticking the pointer in a pocket with easy access will diminish extraneous use of that tool.
- Even if a handheld pointer is available, if there are dual screens, the better option is to use the mouse to point to important information. This way, the "point" will show up on both screens simultaneously and allow engagement with audience members on both sides of the room.

Go Slow on Tables and Figures

One mistake that is often made is to fly through a table or figure during a presentation. Take time to orient the audience to each element of a table or figure before revealing the result of that element. Remember, the audience is not familiar with that element, so if rushed, they will be left wondering what they were even looking at (Sidebar 13-6). Give a chance for audience members to digest the message and meaning.

Answering Questions

Depending on the venue or conference, audience questions might be asked during a presentation or saved for the end. In either case, the speaker should follow what is customary for that particular setting. Before jumping into the answer, repeat the question. Many times, other audience members cannot hear the question that was asked, rendering the answer useless. Further, repeating the question can help ensure that the attendee's question was fully understood. Lastly, repeating the question gives the speaker a couple of moments to collect thoughts and take a breath before launching into the response. As indicated previously, give an honest and complete answer, without rambling too far off topic.

Do Not Go Over the Allotted Time

This is a combination of planning and respect. Exceeding allotted time sends the message that the presentation was not planned or practiced and/or that the speaker does not care, demonstrating disrespect for the audience, the conference organizers, and the subsequent speakers. Plan slides appropriately and practice sufficiently so the total delivery time is known and not exceeded.

Conclusion

Public speaking and presenting can be nerve-racking, especially when the speaker is new to it. However, with careful planning, preparation, and practice, the experience can be less intimidating and even become fun. Review the end of chapter checklists to ensure that the most important points are covered for design (Sidebar 13-7) and delivery (Sidebar 13-8). Enjoy the process by putting a creative and thoughtful stamp in the visuals of the slides, and send a clear and well-developed message. Practice thoughtfully, and find the spaces where there may be pitfalls in the slideshow or in presentation style. Finally, put on a performance with a smooth delivery and, even if nervous, stay confident and in control. Enjoy the show!

Bibliography

Beebe SA, Biggers T. Emotion-eliciting qualities of speech delivery and their effect on credibility and comprehension. Paper presented at: the Annual Meeting of the International Communication Association; May 21-June 2, 1988; New Orleans, LA.

Berk RA. Research on PowerPoint: from basic features to multimedia. *Int J Technol Teaching Learning*. 2011;7(1):24-35.

Berk RA. Top 10 evidence-based, best practices for PowerPoint in the classroom. *Transformative Dialogues: Teaching Learning J*. 2012;5(3):1-7.

Castillo M. Making a point: getting the most out of PowerPoint. *Am J Neuroradiol*. 2011;32(2):217-219.

Collins J. Education techniques for lifelong learning: giving a PowerPoint presentation: the art of communicating effectively. *Radiographics*. 2004;24(4):1185-1192.

Collins J. Education techniques for lifelong learning: making a PowerPoint presentation. *Radiographics*. 2004;24(4):1177-1183.

Daffner RH. On improvement of scientific presentations: using PowerPoint. *Am J Roentgenol*. 2003;181(1):47-49.

De Wet C. Beyond presentations: using PowerPoint as an effective instructional tool. *Gifted Child Today*. 2006;29(4):29-39.

Duarte N. *Slide:ology: The Art and Science o Creating Great Presentations*. Sebastopol, CA: O'Reilly Media; 2008.

Durso FT, Pop VL, Burnett JS, Stearman EJ. Evidence-based human factors guidelines for PowerPoint presentations. *Ergonomics Design*. 2011;19(3):4-8.

Harolds JA. Tips for giving a memorable presentation, part V: stage fright and rehearsing a presentation. *Clin Nucl Med*. 2012;37(11):1094-1096.

James KE, Burke LA, Hutchins HM. Powerful or pointless? Faculty versus student perceptions of PowerPoint use in business education. *Business Communication Q*. 2006;69(4):374-396.

Jones AM. The use and abuse of PowerPoint in teaching and learning in the life sciences: a personal overview. *Biosci Educ*. 2003;2(1):1-13.

Reynolds G. *Presentation Zen Design: Simple Design Principles and Techniques to Enhance Your Presentations*. Berkeley, CA: New Riders; 2010.

Tarpley MJ, Tarpley JL. The basics of PowerPoint and public speaking in medical education. *J Surg Educ*. 2008;65(2):129-132.

Wesner BS, Hynes GE. It's not what you say, it's how you say it...or is it? Elements that business professionals consider most important in speakers. *J Organizational Culture Commun Conflict*. 2015;19(Special Issue):87-96.

Sidebar 13-7

Slideshow Design Checklist
- ☐ Appropriate slide count/number (remember the 67% to 75% rule)
- ☐ Colors (compliment, not clash and ones that can be easily seen)
- ☐ Placeholders and images—size and spacing
- ☐ Minimize the number of words per slide
- ☐ Minimize bullet point use
- ☐ Appropriate font size(s)
- ☐ Use images approximately—borders, pixel size, contribute to the message, coloring

Sidebar 13-8

Presentation Checklist
Before
- ☐ Design a great slideshow
- ☐ Save to thumb drive (or 2!)
- ☐ Email file to yourself (just in case)
- ☐ Contact the event organizer to ensure any audio-visual needs
- ☐ Practice!

On-site
- ☐ Check in with IT personnel
- ☐ Upload presentation and video files, if needed
- ☐ Obtain/ensure internet access, if needed
- ☐ Become familiar with presentation hardware (eg, pointer/slide advancer, mouse, cables to hook into if using you own laptop, where to plug in your own thumb drive, etc)
- ☐ Take a deep breath—you are prepared!

During
- ☐ Set up a timer (your phone or a watch) if there is no clock
- ☐ Say your "thanks"
- ☐ Deliver
- ☐ Answer questions
- ☐ Say "thanks" again, just for good measure

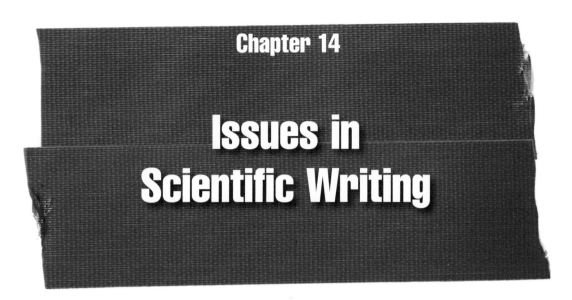

Chapter 14

Issues in Scientific Writing

*Jeff G. Konin, PhD, ATC, PT, FACSM, FNATA
and Elisabeth C. Rosencrum, PhD, NH-LAT, ATC, CSCS*

Much of this textbook addresses scientific and research-oriented approaches toward successful grantsmanship and scholarship. An underlying consideration too often neglected is that of what is known as *authorship*. In simple, unscientific terms, authorship refers to the names of those individuals listed as contributors to a published manuscript. For the sake of this discussion, this chapter will focus its attention to those manuscripts submitted to peer-reviewed journals; albeit, similar concepts of authorship would and should apply to textbook and other writing contributions. Single-authored manuscripts are exempt from this discussion as there are no considerations of author order that would need to be made. Both single author and multiple contributor manuscripts will adhere to the same rules discussed later in this chapter related to issues of plagiarism.

Historically, single author manuscripts have carried a perception of impressive nature. In academic institutions where faculty are considered for promotion and tenure based upon their scholarship production, being a single author has typically served as an admirable accomplishment. Despite much of health care and education being multidisciplinary and interprofessional in nature, only recently has collaborative research and writing gained greater consideration and attention. This shift is likely a result of interprofessional efforts to yield more efficient outcomes.[1] Nonetheless, the collaborative trend in scholarly work has yielded a larger number of multi-authored manuscripts. As a result, each contributor has a vested interest in how his or her name appears in the author order given the attributions associated with institutional and professional publishing expectations.[2]

Authorship

One would think that through centuries of scientific publishing, standards would exist to help guide us on the proper etiquette of authorship. Fortunately, uniform requirements do exist, although they are not necessarily known or adhered to by all. One is more likely to find

Knoblauch M. *Professional Writing in Kinesiology and Sports Medicine* (pp 175-186).
© 2019 Taylor & Francis Group.

established guidelines for authorship in biomedical, social science, and humanities journals.[3] The International Committee of Medical Journal Editors (ICMJE) have set guidelines that journals are encouraged to follow.[1,4,5] In 2016, Resnik et al[3] studied authorship policies of scientific journals and found that only 62.5% of such journals had authorship policies in place. They also reported a positive correlation with having authorship policies and a journal impact factor. This might suggest a greater concern and higher level of importance to identify each author's role with a given manuscript submission and publication. In further analyzing existing journal authorship policies, they found the following items to be addressed:

- Guidance on criteria for authorship = 99.7%
- Guidance on acknowledgments = 97.3%
- Requirement of an authors' substantial contributions to the research = 94.7%
- Requirement of an authors' accountability for the research as a whole = 84.8%
- Guidance on changes in authorship = 77.9%
- Requirements that all authors give final approval of the manuscript = 77.6%
- Requirement that all authors draft or critically revise the manuscript = 71.7%
- Guidance on corporate (collaborative) authorship = 58.9%
- Policy prohibiting gift, guest, or ghost authorship = 31.7%
- Requirement of all authors to describe their contributions = 5.3%
- Limitation on the number of total authors for certain types of articles = 4.0%
- Requirement of each author to be accountable for his or her part of the research = 1.1%

The bottom line is that anyone involved with scientific writing should take the time to learn about recommended guidelines for authorship to avoid potential disputes and conflicts among collaborators.[6]

Order of Authorship

The order in which multi-authored papers are listed can be controversial as there are many ways to approach the decision-making process of determining the order by which contributors are listed. Some methods commonly followed are rooted in tradition in academia and assumptions about authorship. For example, some may subscribe to the notion that the most senior-ranking contributor be listed as first author, regardless of the amount of work he or she has contributed to the manuscript. However, experienced authors know better than to rely on assumptions when it comes to listing authors of a manuscript for final submission. As there are numerous methods of approaching order of authorship, understanding the characters at play can be vital. Senior researchers might not serve as lead authors or primary investigators, but remain involved in the project by supervising the research of junior researchers as is common with graduate student research. In this case, more junior researchers should serve as the first author.

One of the first items that should be addressed prior to establishing authorship order is whether a person is even listed as an author on a paper. In considering this, the best source of reference may be the guidelines recommended by the ICMJE for determining co-authorship.[5] The ICMJE guidelines for co-authorship are as follows.

To be recognized as a co-author, an individual must:

- Contribute significantly to the conception, design, execution, and/or analysis and interpretation of data
- Participate in drafting and/or revising part of the manuscript for intellectual content
- Approve the version to be published
- Agree to be accountable for all aspects of the work

There are 2 ways to approach these 4 criteria. First, be sure that any listed author of a manuscript submission can comfortably and unequivocally state affirmative to each of the criteria. Every listed author must be accountable for all of the subject matter.[1] Second, be sure that anyone else who has been involved with the research and who has also met all of the criteria is not omitted from appropriate authorship.

The first criterion identified by the ICMJE is an area that can be open to discussion and possible disagreement among co-authors. The definition of a "significant contribution" may be viewed differently by each contributor, which could lead to conversations surrounding the perceived role of each. This is especially true if no pre-established agreement regarding each contributor's role and expectations have been made, but it can also be a problem if a pre-established agreement has been made and the interpretation is varied of whether one has fulfilled the agreed-upon obligations. The American Medical Association *Manual of Style* defines *substantial contribution* as an "… important intellectual contribution, without which the work, or an important part of the work, could not have been completed or the manuscript could not have been written or submitted for publication".[7(p128)]

Some would suggest that the senior researcher plays a key role in determining authorship. The senior researcher, listed as the last author, could meet early with potential authors, explain expectations, and educate each person on the specific project and protocol for potential authorship. In many cases, this serves as an effective way to streamline a trusted method of authorship inclusion and order. However, it should be noted that situations do arise where the lead author, and sometimes co-authors as well, raises a concern that the senior researcher has not necessarily met the criteria for inclusion of authorship. This is obviously a concern and also leads to ethical dilemmas, particularly in situations where students serve as the lead researcher and corresponding author. While potentially uncomfortable, it is in everyone's best interest to openly discuss such concerns as soon as possible.

The best advice that can be given is to establish as early as possible who will be considered as a listed contributor for authorship.[6,8] Doing this can avoid uneasy conversations and conflicts at later dates. Agreeing upon authorship roles and responsibilities early can also lead to known accountability for each person throughout the writing process. One thing to recognize is that the order of authorship does not in and of itself define the amount of work that has been contributed by each person. Consider the following:

> *Konin JG, Tawt LP, Harrison BG, Winchester AT. Outcomes assessment of early intervention following acute patella instability.* Inter-Professional Journal of Sports Medicine. *2017;1(1):12-19.*

Four authors contributed to this peer-reviewed published manuscript. Konin is listed as the "first" author, commonly referred to as the *lead author*. For clarification purposes, Tawt is the "second" author, and Winchester is the "last" author. There is no formal term used to describe others listed in the authorship. Therefore, Harrison may be referred to as the "third" author, but typically the first and last author are the ones who might be perceived as having the greatest roles in a manuscript submission. It is important to note, however, that this is not always the case, as is commonly seen with position or consensus statements that may include up to 20 contributing authors. It is not uncommon to see authors listed in alphabetical order when there are large numbers involved with the manuscript.[9]

Most will agree that the lead author is the most involved with the manuscript submission. This individual will accept all of the responsibilities associated with the manuscript. With respect to the submission process, the lead author will typically serve as the person of primary correspondence between the manuscript authors and the journal editor. The lead author will also be responsible for assuring that all of the identified contributors holding authorship complete any required forms for the journal submission in a timely and appropriate manner. The forms may include biography information (credentials, affiliations, contact information), conflicts of interest statements, and acknowledgments of contributions to the manuscript. Without a doubt, the lead author takes on a greater role than other contributors and, as a result, benefits from the authorship order when the manuscript is eventually published by way of first author position recognition.

An individual listed as the last author of a manuscript could in fact bring about a number of inferences. In some cases, multiple authors may list themselves in alphabetical order or in order by which they felt their contributions were put forth. As there is no singular rule on author order, it is not always possible to identify the reason for the order decided upon by the authors of a published manuscript. Individual published manuscripts do not list the process used to determine the order of authorship. However, it is a commonly accepted practice among experienced and well-published scholars to list the senior researcher last. There are a variety of reasons for this rationale. It is possible that the funding to support the research leading to the manuscript submission was obtained by the senior researcher. It is also possible that the author listed last is actually overseeing this project as part of a larger scholarly line of work in his or her lab. Often, the work of graduate students will earn them lead author status on the resulting manuscripts, with their research supervisor listed as last author. In such relationships as those between graduate students and senior researchers/research supervisors, it is acknowledged that the senior researcher plays an important role in the process of publishing an article.[1] This role ranges from conception of the research question to data collection to editing the manuscript for proper factual content and the avoidance of plagiarism. For example, does the placement of authorship determine who is responsible for coordinating the manuscript submission? There is no correct answer to this as it simply resorts to the clear communication among contributors preferably accomplished early in the process.

An example of a situation where the senior researcher may come into question regarding authorship can be recognized in this vignette:

> Maren is a PhD student who recently successfully defended her dissertation. Her advisor, Dr. Bryan, is a well-known expert in the kinesiology field. He has to his credit over 100 peer-reviewed manuscripts, has obtained numerous National Institutes of Health grants, is a highly sought-after speaker at professional conferences, and has mentored many graduate students over his lengthy and successful academic career at a highly reputable Carnegie Research I University. Following her formal graduation, Maren accepted a position as a junior faculty member at a small liberal arts university. As part of her scholarly agenda planning, she spent some time sifting through the large data sets collected from her doctoral work and realized that she is able to answer an important question and submit a manuscript on this finding. In doing so, she reaches out to Dr. Bryan for his collaborative involvement. Dr. Bryan takes 1 to 2 weeks to respond to each of her emails with very brief responses that Maren struggles to find helpful. After Maren drafts a manuscript for submission, she seeks Dr. Bryan's feedback and expertise with editing the work. Despite numerous email and telephone prompts, she never hears back or receives feedback from Dr. Bryan. At this point, Maren opts to submit the manuscript to a peer-reviewed journal and, in doing so, makes the difficult decision of not putting Dr. Bryan's name on the paper as an author. Instead, she acknowledges his advisory role with data collection while she was a doctoral student in his research lab. With some small revisions, Maren's paper is accepted and soon after published. Upon publication, Dr. Bryan becomes aware of the paper, and becomes infuriated that he is not listed as a formal author.

Was Maren's decision making sound? Should Maren have done anything differently to attract Dr. Bryan's attention to the manuscript and/or confirm his appropriate involvement or noninterest to participate? Appropriate building of relationships can alleviate many of these communication difficulties. Having not only pre-established guidelines but also an open and communicative relationship helps to avoid situations like Maren's. This example is not uncommon, and it can be avoided. In this particular case, one might believe that Maren made every effort to do the right thing, yet as a result of her decision, she has likely ended any chance of a continued professional collegial relationship with her research mentor, Dr. Bryan.

Would it have been appropriate for Maren to list Dr. Bryan as an author on this manuscript even though he did not contribute in any way? If she did, how would she have provided signed documents on his behalf confirming his complete involvement according to the ICMJE guidelines? Regardless of what Maren chose to do, she should be sure to take into account all of the ethical, legal, and even political considerations prior to moving forward. In this case, what would happen if Dr. Bryan contacted the journal and placed a complaint that he was omitted from being recognized as an author? Journals do not choose to participate in accepting the responsibility of such conflicts, which is why they require authors to sign acknowledgment of their work as a contributor. Journals have no way of knowing if an author was omitted from being listed on a paper. However, authors who sign an acknowledgment that they, in fact, met all of the criteria for being listed hold themselves accountable to the appropriate ethical expectations of authorship. Again, a journal is in no way responsible for knowing or proving if an author has falsified his or her statement. For these reasons, it is always best to handle authorship considerations between the potential authors and contributors. If authors are not able to agree on inclusion or order, they should consult with administrators at their own institutions as well as other respected professionals who can provide an objective opinion on one's involvement or lack thereof.

Ethics of Author Inclusion and Exclusion

The reality of scientific publishing is that there are circumstances where individuals are included as authors despite not having met the appropriate inclusion criteria, and yet others may be omitted when they should have been included based on their role in the overall workload. These situations are far too common, and it is important to outline those situations that lead to their occurrence.

Guest authorship, otherwise known as *honorary authorship*, occurs when individuals are assigned authorship but have not met the previously stated authorship criteria. Guest authors may have not contributed substantially to the work.[10] As described earlier, guest authorship is not an uncommon practice and may be prominent in academic environments. In the case of Maren and Dr. Bryan, had Maren included him on the manuscript submission, he truly would be classified as a guest author. Guest authorship has also been granted to department chairs and deans, which would be inappropriate if their only role was that of general supervision.[11]

Guest authorship may be utilized for a number of reasons, but there are other options as well. In some cases, authors will recruit others to serve in a guest role for the purposes of increasing the chances of journal acceptance.[10] Junior scholars may partner with a recognized leader in the field who only serves to assist from a peripheral distance. In this case, the guest may assist with manuscript preparation but has never been directly involved in the data collection. Other times, an author may not be successful in achieving journal acceptance, having already been rejected. Reaching out to a more experienced scholar may assist in revising the manuscript and improving one's chances of journal acceptance. However, in such a case, the added individuals should more than likely not be listed as an author having not met all of the authorship criteria. Instead, being *acknowledged* in the manuscript would be the correct approach. When guest authors are included and formally recognized on a published paper, it has the potential of devaluing the work of the other authors since the true validity of contributions has been impacted.[2]

Technically speaking, any person what has contributed to the manuscript but has not been able to meet the criteria for authorship should be acknowledged. Observationally, one might conjecture that acknowledgments have been reserved for those who have assisted with typesetting, recruitment of subjects, loaning of equipment or space, or other tasks related to the ability to complete a research project. While this is the case most times, and deservedly so, an acknowledgment should also be reserved for individuals who have assisted with the manuscript preparation but who have not met all of the ICMJE criteria to earn authorship. As a result of guest authorship practices, too many authors have been liberal in their inclusiveness of full authorship recognition vs an appropriate acknowledgment. Whether it is considered as a kind gesture of one's appreciation for an individual's assistance with the manuscript or the understanding that all contributors would prefer authorship credit for their own dossier, it is not ethically acceptable.

Ghost authors are another form of authorship that may raise concern. Ghost authors actually contribute in a substantial manner to a manuscript yet are not even acknowledged. Consider an author who is struggling to have a manuscript accepted by a journal. The author seeks the assistance of a senior researcher, who in return not only offers some advice, but makes some edits and essentially rewrites the manuscript to an extent whereby it eventually receives journal acceptance. The senior researcher clearly does not warrant full authorship as all 4 ICJME requirements were not met, even though full authorship may have been offered by the original author as an act of kindness. More so, the senior researcher requests not to receive any credit whatsoever for the act of "helping out." However, without proper acknowledgment of the senior researcher's assistance, there is a lack of transparency and accountability demonstrated on the part of the original author by adding on a ghostwriter at a later phase.[8,10] In this example, the original author is essentially accepting full credit for the work published since journal reviewers and editors, and, ultimately, readers of the literature, will have no idea of any ghostwriting that has occurred.

The practice of ghostwriting is believed to date back to the early 1900s and is actually considered acceptable by some journals and medical schools. However, many consider this to be a form of plagiarism and criticize the process. It has been estimated that between 4.9% and 16.2% of peer-reviewed manuscripts employ ghostwriters.[12] Medical writers (those that simply edit for grammar and technical writing) are not considered ghostwriters, although they may certainly be formally acknowledged if an author chooses to do so.[13]

One final point to consider with respect to the disclosure of authorship is that of potential conflicts of interest. Accompanying a manuscript submission, and certainly with an accepted and published manuscript, full acknowledgment of any potential conflicts of interest must be disclosed by each author and anyone else responsible for the completion of the research and paper. Conflicts of interest may include, but are not limited to, the following:

- Financial relationships supporting the research (honorariums, stock ownership, product or equipment arrangements, patent ownership)
- Employment relationships associated with the research (receiving payment for direct work functions)
- Consultation relationships associated with the research (receiving a stipend as a consultant)
- Maintaining a personal relationship with a biased influence to produce desired positive outcomes

When a conflict of interest is disclosed, some journals will simply state their policy and decision not to review or accept the submitted manuscript up front. However, not all disclosed potential conflicts of interest result in a manuscript not being reviewed. The nature of the reported conflict is reviewed and, if accepted, it is clearly stated if the manuscript results in publication. It should be noted, however, that others could perceive the results of a study as being biased despite the journal agreeing to publication. It is always best to carefully review journal policies prior to submission for potential conflicts (see Chapter 6 for more information about journal policies), and to self-assess one's decision-making process when planning a study that could pose a conflict of interest.

Potential conflicts of interest may arise when relationships between researchers and product development occur. It is common for researchers to study new products affiliated with third-party companies. These companies look for studies that demonstrate positive outcomes associated with their product. When doing so, it is important to enter into agreements with companies carefully to avoid inadvertent and/or unethical reported findings related to research funding and support. The development of a written contractual agreement can be helpful. This document should state the terms of the study, clearly defining the role of the researchers, data being collected, and dissemination of the results of the findings.

Researchers who choose to test a product owned by a third-party company should do so without accepting any form of compensation paid directly to the researcher for the purpose of product outcomes. The product itself is typically provided by the company at no cost, and it is possible that fees necessary to perform the testing, such as for space, research assistants, university overhead, etc can be funded. However, all researchers should be careful to assure that there is no personal financial benefit, or other personal quid pro quo–type relationship that exists with the agreement to test a product. Personal financial gain for the researcher will ultimately taint the results as personal profit could potentially influence the study's results and, in the long run, have a negative impact on both the researcher's reputation and the potential benefit of the product being tested.

While a company that owns a product will want to possess data collected from research of said product, any researcher entering into an agreement to test a product with a third party should clearly agree to ownership of the data. This is typical protocol and will likely be verified by an organization's institutional review board prior to collecting the data. Furthermore, the researcher should assure in writing that he or she has a scholarly obligation to publish the results as found. In an effort to avoid demonstration of the data in an inaccurately positive light, the researcher should maintain neutrality in analysis and presentation of the data.

Appropriate Citation

When setting out to submit a written work, there are many recommendations that may vary depending on the journal, publisher, editors, etc. An example of such was the advice given to the contributors of this text by way of publisher guidelines. One of the guidelines read as follows:

> *Ensure that your writing is original, does not exist in the public domain, does not violate the right of privacy of any person, and is not libelous or obscene and does not infringe upon the statutory or common copyright of anyone.*

Essentially, the publisher is saying **do not plagiarize**.

Plagiarism may be the single greatest ethical violation associated with scientific research. Even in the construction of this text, awareness and prevention of plagiarism has been at the forefront of the development process. In the guidelines sent to chapter contributors, it was clear that originality in content and proper crediting of sources were major concerns. When egregious, it could have legal implications. Plagiarism has been defined by the Office of Research Integrity as "Theft or misappropriation of intellectual property and the substantial unattributed textual copying of another's work."[14(p77)] More simply put, plagiarism consists of stealing written intellectual information from others and can include, but is not limited to, another person's ideas, methodology, results and findings, or a complete usage of words or phrases without giving proper credit to the owner of the work. Plagiarism may also include photos, tables, and figures belonging to others.

One would assume that the majority of authors do not intentionally plagiarize their work. However, there has recently been a noted increase of plagiarism within the scientific literature.[15] Why would one intentionally plagiarize? As discussed previously, there are enormous pressures to publish scholarly work if an individual is employed in a setting where scholarship is the main attribute associated with professional promotion.[14] Additionally, there is a trend for journals to favor manuscripts that have demonstrated statistical significance as well as findings that reveal something of clinical importance. Conducting research and preparing a manuscript can be very time consuming. In the absence of significant findings, an author knows that publication may not be possible, hence the pressure to manipulate the findings to reveal a different result.[16] Such research misconduct has been reported by Juyal[14] to include falsification of the process to include the reporting of fabricated results. In the end, the responsibility for ethical research conduct and truthful conclusions belongs to the authors.[13] However, journals have a heightened awareness of scrutiny as they will entertain the backlash of a poor reputation if they become known for repeated publication of plagiarized work.

A known plagiarized, published manuscript can end up being retracted, though this is not the most common reason for publication retraction. Plagiarism accounts for some 32% of retracted manuscripts.[17] Other reasons for manuscript retraction include various forms of identified misconduct, errors in data calculations, and possible found redundancy of the manuscript with another journal.

To make maximal efforts for avoiding plagiarism, Debnath[18] suggests the following:

- Increase awareness and education of ethical research conduct.
- Follow clear and definitive established policies.
- Use an author certificate (or disclaimer) stating copyright integrity.
- Use software for plagiarism checks.

Plagiarism can be found in many forms. Surprisingly, one of the more commonly seen forms is referred to as *unconscious plagiarism*. Unconscious plagiarism is simply not being aware of what does and does not constitute plagiarism. Such information is typically taught in an introduction to research methods class that addresses ethics associated with research. However, unconscious plagiarism has also been associated with poor writing skills.[15] In a 2017 study of second-year medical students in Romania, a large percentage of students reported a lack of understanding that simply changing words does not avoid plagiarism.[19] With young investigators, a common concern seen is that of not knowing what is considered to be common knowledge within a designated specialty. After all, it takes a reasonably long time for one to become familiar with a majority of the published work, especially those manuscripts of historical significance. Young investigators likely do not possess such accessible knowledge and now live in an era of information explosion. As a result, manuscripts may include information that is not properly attributed to a source but instead may seem to be common knowledge by an author. One of the more important roles of a senior researcher and mentor is to guide a young investigator away from this error.

Cultural differences can result in tensions from plagiarism as well. In many other cultures, it is customary in the educational systems to recite verbatim the words of educators or texts as a sign of respect.[20] This practice persisting to publication can be problematic, especially crossing cultural differences in proper crediting for original work done. Imagine an author reaches publication of their work only to find another piece years later with blatantly plagiarized content. From a Western perspective, this could certainly be infuriating; feeling ownership of original content only to see it used without reference to your work. Culturally, such a situation should be handled with care.

Cultural differences in tolerance for academic dishonesty have been well documented. Among cultures examined, students in the United States have been found to be the least tolerant of plagiarism and other dishonest academic practices.[21] Academics in some regions have even recognized the troublesome nature of plagiarism but have failed to recognize its presence in their practice. In some Latin American regions, for example, inconsistencies in the application of plagiarism have been noted as a concern. Plagiarism in writing without attributing the source was seen as less problematic than the inappropriate use of original data; however, few standards and practices are in place to combat the issue.[22] As scholars in a field with much content and application crossover and international relevance, the recognition and handling of cultural differences in plagiarism must be carefully approached.

Inappropriate referencing is another form of plagiarism. Though it may not be intentional in all cases, it does fall short of ethical standards. Content within a manuscript that has been obtained from another source and is not referenced or does not provide proper credit is a form of inappropriate referencing. Some consider secondary reference use a form of plagiarism. A secondary reference is one that is cited by an author in a body of work without going back to the original source. When one reviews that body of work and chooses to use the content in a new manuscript, the original source should be cited, not the secondary source where the information was found.

For example, when reading a textbook to learn about meniscal special tests, a researcher comes across one of the citations that is a published systematic review of all special tests for the knee. The textbook itself does a nice job of summarizing the systematic review paper. The researcher then drafts a paper and cites the textbook as its source for the information obtained. Technically, the textbook is a secondary reference for the content of the systematic review, and it is the original systematic review paper that should be cited. This obviously requires that the researcher track down that paper and review it for him- or herself. Furthermore, paraphrasing from the textbook could potentially be another form of plagiarism as previously discussed. Secondary references are used sparingly and, in particular, when an original source is no longer in print and is unattainable.

Another common mistake associated with plagiarism occurs with citing textbooks as reference sources. It should never be assumed or guaranteed that when authors update textbook editions, they only add information that is more current. Many times, information is also deleted that has become obsolete or no longer of relevance to the textbook. Therefore, when one finds information in a textbook that is used for a citation, a search should always be performed to learn if the textbook has a more current edition in print. If so, the current edition must be reviewed and verified for the presence of the content of interest to be cited. If the content has been removed, it is not appropriate to cite the older edition of the text as it will be out of print and unavailable to the potential reader. This also holds true for using any textbook as a citation if it is no longer in print (ie, published copy). One would need to locate the information from a different source.

Perhaps the most obvious form of plagiarism is when one literally copies word-for-word someone else's published and copyrighted work. Doing so is unethical, even if the copied material is cited as is. If it is cited as is, it must be in parentheses and clearly noted that the work is paraphrased and belongs to someone else. What is referred to as a *cut-and-paste* without any citation is unfortunately a simple and common method of plagiarism. This insinuates that the work is of one's own when, in fact, it truly belongs to someone else. The expanded use of computers has been a contributor to the ease of accessibility to cut-and-paste existing copyrighted work that is displayed as one's own. In some cases, this has been referred to as *redundant publication*.[23] With redundant publication, similar content in reasonable amounts are submitted in more than one manuscript without acknowledging the identical work elsewhere. This is similar to what is referred to as *text recycling*, where portions of text from a previously published manuscript are used without appropriate citation and/or permission.

Masic et al[24] predict that problems of plagiarism will become the most discussed topic of the modern scientific world due to the development of standard measures to rank an author's work. Nowadays, it has become best practice for both students and faculty alike to utilize software programs to detect plagiarism.[15,24] Zhang[25] also recommends the use of workflow processes to avoid plagiarism. It is beyond the scope of this chapter to discuss the various vendors and plagiarism detection software programs that are currently on the market as technology will likely change at a rapid pace and result in more sophisticated and a greater number of programs in years to come. However, readily available programs do currently exist, and some studies have been performed to guide researchers on the use of plagiarism avoidance via software detection. Zhang and Jia[26] performed a study that was commissioned by the Committee on Publication Ethics and made recommendations based upon similarity indexes that can be utilized. Similarity indexes are identified by the software as a way of reporting how much of a manuscript matches wording and phrasing of existing published and copyrighted work. The authors actually suggested a similarity index of 30 (ie, 30% similarity between 2 works) as the cut-off point of concern. While 30% similarity is the standard suggested by the authors, other senior researchers may feel as though 30% similarity is too high and would raise concern.

One last form of plagiarism worth discussing is that of "self-plagiarism." Self-plagiarism is also referred to as *salami slicing*.[27,28] Fonseca[29] defined salami slicing as "the practice of partitioning a large study that could have been reported in a single research article into smaller published articles." What does this mean? Instead of submitting one's work as a single large data set as part of a manuscript, the data set is "sliced" into multiple sets and results in a few smaller studies. With publication, this may be observed as part I and II when, in fact, there is no reason it could not have been a single publication.[30,31] By some, this is considered to be unethical. To be clear, it is not unethical if the original data set is extremely large. In many cases, large data sets are collected over years, yielding different findings at various points in time. This is seen commonly with population-based data collection. In such cases, the key is to assure that each paper is truly distinct from the other and answers a different research question.[29] Salami slicing is also found where individuals slightly revise a published manuscript and submit it to a second journal that published its work in a different language. When this is done, it is not likely to be recognized and may pass through the editors' review undetected.

Why would one partake in this behavior if it may be considered unethical? Again, the pressure to publish is faced by many researchers and faculty. Salami slicing allows for a greater number of peer-reviewed publications and will yield increased quantity while not necessarily detracting from the quality of a single paper. It is quite possible that even though a single large paper is split in 2, the quality of both papers is still respectable. It is a reasonable assumption that a greater number of published manuscripts will yield a greater number of citations by others, thus referring to the ranking of one's overall body of work. In most institutions, aside from the consideration of a journal impact factor, a greater number of publications and citations will support an individual's career pathway to successful and possibly faster promotion. This does not only pertain to faculty and other researchers as both master and doctoral level candidates also feel pressures of launching a scholarly career and the need to publish peer-reviewed research.[16,32]

Conclusion

Scholarship is associated with many aspects of appropriate preparation and submission. Authorship is one consideration that is often overlooked yet plays a key role in proper identification of one's contribution to a research project and manuscript. Authorship order and the identification of author's contributions are important components that should be clearly identified early on in the research process. Other forms of acknowledgment exist and should be utilized appropriately in accordance with one's contribution. Understanding research ethics and the various forms of plagiarism are also key factors to be cognizant of as they pertain to manuscript submission. The lead author and/or senior researcher play vital roles and take on the responsibility and accountability to assure that no form of plagiarism is found with a manuscript submission.

Case Scenarios

Authorship Order Based on Contributions: Case #1—Divide and Conquer

Suzanne, Edith, and Tom were all doctoral students together in overlapping cohorts at a small college. Under the guidance and support of their program director, they designed and collected data for a project unrelated to their dissertations. Since completing their doctoral studies and establishing themselves as junior faculty members at their respective institutions, they have decided to revisit the project for the purpose of publication.

Suzanne, Edith, and Tom begin planning their division of duties. They decide due to workload and expectations for tenure at their respective institutions that Suzanne and Edith will take the lead in developing the content for the article. They decide as a group that Tom will serve in more of an editorial role, checking their study design, triangulating data, and fixing any technical writing issues. Their program director mentor supports their work but continues to have very little active role in the production of the published work.

Case #1 Questions for Discussion

- In what order should the authors be listed? Why?
- What type of authorship should be granted to each? Why?
- Should Tom still be considered an author? Why or why not?

Plagiarism: Case #2—Other Languages Are Hard

Amaya completed a qualitative study using an inductive approach in which she used a unique data analysis method that is uncommon in the literature. Amaya discovered the method of analysis in an article that had been translated to English from a foreign language. The translation revealed nomenclature that resembled another qualitative approach that was not used in Amaya's study.

Amaya properly cited the source and appropriately described and utilized the technique in her study. Upon submission for review, reviewers became confused about the technique Amaya used, stating that she did not appropriately reference the original work in which the technique appeared. Amaya is concerned because she did not use the method the reviewers are concerned with, and she absolutely does not want to be flagged as plagiarizing in her work.

Case #2 Questions for Discussion

- Did Amaya plagiarize?
- How can Amaya clarify the methods she used in her study?
- What can the reviewers do to communicate, clarify, or communicate the issue to Amaya?

Decision Making to Publish Based Upon Journal Rating and Perception: Case #3—Something Better Than Nothing

Brent is a new junior faculty member and begins to work toward publication of portions of his dissertation. Brent has several components of his dissertation that are worthy of publication, and he would like to start with submitting some of the easier, more basic content. In the process of deciding how to focus his publication energies, Brent decides to submit the most basic portion of his dissertation for publication in a regional, "lower-level" journal and save the more authentic, groundbreaking portions of his study for larger, more respected journals.

The journal has only 1 year of quarterly editions published, and the editors are eager to have more versions filled, leading the faculty member to believe it may be easier to have his paper accepted. Brent works at an institution that is not "publish or perish," but he needs some scholarly activity for his mid-tenure review.

Case #3 Questions for Discussion

- How is Brent's thought process? Does his decision make sense?
- Will his publication in the lower-level journal be of value to him?
- What factors should Brent weigh when making a decision like this?

References

1. Shemer A, Shoenfeld Y. Authorship—a great honor or an onerous responsibility? *Harefuah*. 2017;1:363-364.
2. Kornhaber RA, McLean LM, Baber RJ. Ongoing ethical issues concerning authorship in biomedical journals: an integrative review. *Int J Nanomedicine*. 2015;10:4837-4846.
3. Resnik DB, Tyler AM, Black JR, Kissling G. Authorship policies of scientific journals. *J Med Ethics*. 2016;42(3);199-202.
4. International Committee of Medical Journal Editors. Author responsibilities—conflicts of interest. http://www.icmje.org/recommendations/browse/roles-and-responsibilities/author-responsibilities--conflicts-of-interest.html. Accessed July 31, 2017.
5. International Committee of Medical Journal Editors. Defining the role of authors and contributors. http://www.icmje.org/recommendations/browse/roles-and-responsibilities/defining-the-role-of-authors-and-contributors.html. Accessed July 31, 2017.
6. Anstey A. Authorship issues: grizzlies, guests and ghosts. *Br J Derm*. 2014;170(6):1209-1210.
7. American Medical Association. *AMA Manual of Style: A Guide for Authors*. 10th ed. New York, NY: Oxford University Press; 2007.
8. Albert T. Eight questions to ask before writing an article. *Br J Hosp Med (Lond)*. 2017;78(6);341-343.
9. Smith E, Williams-Jones B. Authorship and responsibility in health sciences research: a review of procedures for fairly allocating authorship in multi-author studies. *Sci Eng Eth*. 2012;18(2):199-212.
10. Citrome L. Authorship: musings about guests and ghosts. *Int J Clin Pract*. 2017;71(7):e12986.
11. Roulet JF. Ethics in publishing. *J Adhes Dent*. 2011;13(1):3.
12. Wilson D, Singer N. Ghostwriting is called rife in medical journals. *New York Times*. September, 10 2009. http://www.nytimes.com/2009/09/11/business/11ghost.html. Accessed July 31, 2017.
13. Matlas-Guiu J, Garcia-Ramos R. Ghost-authors, improvement article communication, and medical publications. *Neurologia*. 2001;26(5):257-261.
14. Juyal D, Thawani V, Thaledi S. Plagiarism: an egregious form of misconduct. *N Am J Med Sci*. 2015;7(2):77-80.
15. Guraya SY, Guraya SS. The confounding factors leading to plagiarism in academic writing and some suggested remedies: a systematic review. *J Pak Med Assoc*. 2017;67(5):767-772.
16. Asghari MH, Moloudizargari M, Abdollahi M. Misconduct in research and publication: a dilemma that is taking place. *Iran Biomed J*. 2017;21(4):203-204.
17. Rai R, Sabharwal S. Retracted publications in orthopaedics: prevalence, characteristics, and trends. *J Bone Joint Surg Am*. 2017;99(9);e44.
18. Debnath J. Letter to the editor: plagiarism in scientific writings: is there any way out? *J Korean Med*. 2017;32(8):1377-1378.
19. Badea O. Do medical students really understand plagiarism? Case study. *Rom J Morphol Embryol*. 2017;58(1):293-296.
20. Redden E. Cheating across cultures. Inside Higher Ed Web site. https://www.insidehighered.com/news/2007/05/24/cheating. Accessed August, 20, 2017.
21. Heitman E, Litewka S. International perspectives on plagiarism and considerations for teaching international trainees. *Urol Oncol*. 2011;29(1):104-108. doi: 10.1016/j.urolonc.2010.09.014.
22. Vasconcelos S, Leta J, Costa L, Pinto A, Sorenson MM. Discussing plagiarism in Latin America. *EMBO Repts*. 2009;4:677-682.
23. Wager E. Why is redundant publication a problem? *Int J Occup Environ Med*. 2015:6(1):3-6.
24. Masic I, Begic E, Dobraca A. Plagiarism detection by online solutions. *Stud Health Technol Inform*. 2017;238:227-230.
25. Zhang YH. CrossCheck: an effective tool for detecting plagiarism. *Learned Publishing*. 2012;23(1):9-14.
26. Zhang YH, Zia XY. A survey on the use of CrossCheck for detecting plagiarism in journal articles. *Learned Publishing*. 2012;25(4):292-307.
27. Rogers LF. From the editor's notebook: salami slicing, shotgunning, and the ethics of authorship. *AJR Am J Roentgenol*. 1999;173(2):265-266.
28. Speilmans GA, Biehn TL, Sawrey DL. A case study of salami slicing: pooled analysis of duloxetine for depression. *Psychother Psychosom*. 2010;79(2):97-106.
29. Fonseca M. The pitfalls of "salami slicing": focus on quality and not quantity of publications. Editage Insights WEb site. http://www.editage.com/insights/the-pitfalls-of-salami-slicing-focus-on-quality-and-not-quantity-of-publications?access-denied-content=metered&InsightsReferer=http://www.editage.com/insights/the-pitfalls-of-salami-slicing-focus-on-quality-and-not-quantity-of-publications?regid=1501182650. Published November 4, 2013. Accessed July 31, 2017.
30. Joob B, Wiwanitkit V. Salami slicing od data set, translational plagiarism, and self-plagiarism: the storyline. *Indian J Psychol Med*. 2017;39(2):218.
31. Menon V, Muraleedharan A. Salami slicing of data sets: what the young researcher needs to know. *Indian J Psychol Med*. 2016;38:577-578.
32. Barbour V. Perverse incentives and perverse publishing practices. *Science Bulletin*. 2015;60:1225-1226.

Chapter 15

Easing the Stress of Writing

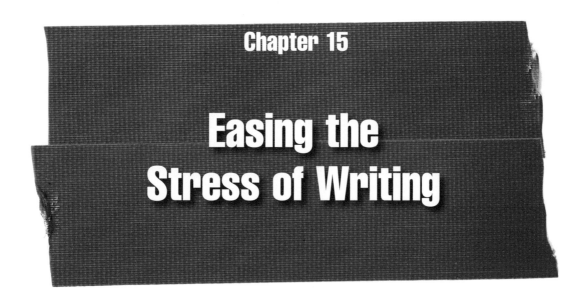

Luzita Vela, PhD, LAT, ATC

At various stages in an academic or professional career, a student or professional may be asked to develop a piece of writing. Some common examples of student writing assignments include literature reviews, evidence-based critiques, abstracts, or a thesis. Similarly, professionals may have to develop a proposal, business letter, or a white paper. The common thread that ties these writing projects together is that they are developed for a purpose: to form a concise, yet clearly articulated, persuasive narrative. The very nature of these assignments not only requires adeptness with the subject matter, but also requires that the student or professional has skills with technical writing.

Interestingly, upon being faced with a writing deadline, one can easily feel overwhelmed by the task, which produces stress. The reason why a person may feel overwhelmed by the task can vary largely from person to person and may include circumstances such as time constraints or having negative previous experiences with writing. This, in turn, influences a person's perceived value of and motivation to complete the project. For example, a student may thumb through a syllabus to be met with an unfortunate sense of dread upon finding that a comprehensive literature review is due at the end of the semester. The student's question that follows is often, "How long does it need to be?" A question such as this indicates that he or she either does not see value in the task or is concerned with his or her own competence to achieve the task. Similarly, a professional may want to make the case to an administrator for additional funding and is told that he or she should develop a proposal with a budget. The automatic response may be to say, "Can't I just talk to you about it?" In this case, the professional may not be able to see how he or she can fit yet another task into his or her busy day-to-day schedule (Sidebar 15-1).

In all of these examples, the affected person may feel that his or her stress is off the charts with the associated stress responses mobilizing at DEFCON 1 levels. Regardless of the underlying cause(s) of the writing stress, there are some ways in which a writer can wrestle back some control and successfully complete the task. This chapter is designed to identify writing motivation techniques and to provide some insight into developing writing practices that are sustainable and effective. Thus, this chapter is organized into 3 sections: the science of writing motivation, writing as a process, and planning and organizing.

Knoblauch M. *Professional Writing in
Kinesiology and Sports Medicine* (pp 187-195).
© 2019 Taylor & Francis Group.

Sidebar 15-1

I had the personal experience where I took a graduate writing class in which I was expected to share my writing with others on a weekly basis. I specifically took the class because I knew that I had deficiencies in my writing, and I automatically feared the judgment of others in the class. Would they all find out I was a fraud and really did not belong in graduate school? Interestingly, I sought out a class to help me feel more comfortable with writing, but to improve my writing, I was required to do the most uncomfortable thing possible, which was share my writing with others. It turned out to be the best experience that I have had with a writing course. Being asked to share writing in a safe environment allowed me to accept the constructive criticism that I received and required me to go back and make edits as part of the process of writing. My writing skills have improved now, not because I have the ability to write better sentences on the first try, but because I realized that all writing work should have several iterations to ensure that the message that was intended to be conveyed is actually understood by the reader. I am now a huge advocate of writing groups and writing assignments with peer feedback.

Finding Writing Motivation

Motivation is a domain-specific characteristic, meaning that whether a person is motivated to complete a task may be influenced by the type of task that he or she is trying to complete.[1,2] A writer may have experienced that feeling where he or she is particularly motivated to complete one assignment while not particularly motivated to complete another. Positive motivation to complete a task matters because it is associated with strategic behavior and task persistence. This is a very important concept because, as the next section will detail, good writing requires a strategic process to be done efficiently and effectively. Achievement motivation is largely affected by self-efficacy beliefs, goals orientation, and personal interests and values.[1] This section will give an overview on how understanding these constructs may provide some ways to positively influence writing motivation.

Self-efficacy is a person's own competence to perform a task and is influenced by both outcomes and efficacy expectations.[1] A person with a good outcomes expectation for writing believes that a particular set of actions will lead to a positive outcome.[2] A positive outcome may be receiving an "A" on a term paper or having a manuscript accepted for publication. Similarly, a person with positive efficacy expectations believes that he or she is actually capable of performing the actions to achieve his or her writing goals. Interestingly, a person may have positive outcomes expectations and believe that setting aside time daily to write is a positive action that will result in better writing. However, the same person may not feel that he or she is capable of creating sustainable writing habits, thus, having negative efficacy expectations. Writing-related self-efficacy evolves over time and may be tied to past success with writing, perceived difficulty of the writing assignment, and perceived effort required for the writing task. For example, a person may have low outcomes beliefs and efficacy beliefs about scientific writing because he or she has had very few positive experiences with scientific writing. Low writing self-efficacy may then result in a writer who feels anxious, avoids help seeking behaviors, or engages in learned helplessness.

Luckily, writing self-efficacy can be influenced. First, novice writers should find a mentor with positive writing motivation. Such mentors can often model coping tactics when faced with a writing challenge. Meaningful ways to engage a mentor include having regularly scheduled meetings to discuss writing challenges, particularly regarding feedback. For example, the peer-review process can be especially challenging to a novice researcher's sense of self-efficacy. A mentor can be helpful in providing perspective and a path to forge forward in the revision process. As such, authors may wish to seek out a mentor and ask if the mentor would be willing to meet periodically to discuss writing challenges.

Next, the writer should think of all writing as developmental to help shift perspective about scientific writing. As with anything else in life, scientific writing improves with practice. Therefore, a writer should celebrate the successes of each part of the writing process, no matter how small. More importantly, writers should recognize that the process for completing the final writing product is composed of small, doable challenges. This shift in perspective can help the writer feel that he or she is in control and can improve feelings regarding writing efficacy. To make the challenges feel attainable, be sure to set realistic writing goals as part of the planning process.

Another good strategy is to view each writing project as a way of developing mastery in a subject matter or in communicating valuable information.[1,2] This way of developing goals for the writing project is termed a *mastery goals approach*, and the focus is on gaining knowledge and improving competence. Using a mastery goals approach recognizes the overall importance of the writing project to one's professional development and can shift how a writer thinks, feels, and engages in the task. For example, in most jobs, communication is a critical task required to be successful. Using a mastery goals approach recognizes that a writing project helps the writer to develop mastery in communication, thus, helping him or her in future professional endeavors. If seen from a larger perspective, a writer is more likely to understand the importance of the writing project, engage in the writing task, and maintain a positive attitude about the project.

Writing Is a Process

Writing Habits

Contrary to what one might see in movies, writing to complete a scientific writing product will rarely be completed in one sitting as a writer is seized by a moment of inspiration. In fact, those who do procrastinate and wait until the last minute to complete a writing project may be able to turn in a completed product, but these products are rarely done well. The simple fact is that successful writing is built as a habit. Most successful scientific writers make the writing process look easy, but this is because they developed writing habits that work for them. For some writers, this means blocking out 1 hour per day to write. Others might find that they prefer to work in larger quantities of time and may block off 2 to 3 hours several times per week to write. The point is that writing is scheduled. Like any habit that we want to reinforce, it should be placed into a calendar and safeguarded from interruptions by other activities.

To feed the writing habit, a writer also needs to consider ways to avoid self-sabotage. Two common forms of self-sabotage are influenced by environment and timing. Finding the right environment that is most conducive for writing is different for each individual. Once the right environment is identified, be sure that the environment is similar each time. This may even change from task to task. For example, a writer might find that, during the early stages of writing, he or she may need longer blocks of time in an environment that is free of all distractions. However, the same writer may find that the editing process can be done in shorter blocks of time in an environment with ambient noise. Writing effectiveness can also be influenced by timing. Some writers may find that they work best first thing in the morning upon waking, while others may prefer writing in the afternoon or evening. Identify patterns of when writing is done most effectively and be sure to block out the same time of day to maximize the time spent on completing writing tasks.

Outline and Zero Draft

A good place to start organizing a writing project is to create an outline. An outline helps to organize the topics that will be covered within the writing project and is a useful tool to structure the way in which a reader will be introduced to various interrelated ideas (see Chapter 2 for more details on creating an outline). A common stressor that occurs after completing an outline is writer's block. A writer may know what he or she wants to write about but does not know how to start. One helpful tool is to use a "zero draft" approach.[3] It is termed a *zero draft* because the end product evolves into a first draft of a paper. A zero draft is a free-writing thought exercise where the writer endeavors to assemble his or her thoughts on the research topic by writing continuously for a set period of time. In a zero draft, the writer does not concern him- or herself with grammar or creating a structured narrative with a thesis statement, complete sentences, and paragraph transitions. In fact, the writer should go against the urge to revise the writing within a zero draft since the revision process interrupts the writer's flow of thoughts. Rather, the writer can use the free-writing exercise to place his or her thoughts on paper. These thoughts are influenced by readings, reflections, and continued questions about the research topic. During the free write, the writer should also not concern him- or herself with providing facts or statistics if they are not known. Instead, the writer can simply state "provide supporting statistic" or "find reference" within the free write (Sidebar 15-2).

Note that the zero draft uses a conversational tone that mimics how a person may think or holds a conversation. Also notice that there are several times where the zero draft says "cite reference," "investigate further," or "stuck here." These are placeholders that indicate that the writer will need to go back and fill in gaps. The product of the next iteration within the writing process is the first draft. Within the first draft, the conversational tone used in the zero draft is changed to fit a scientific writing tone. In addition, areas are expanded upon and transitions are added.

The zero draft can be effective for a person who feels overwhelmed by the idea of starting the process of writing. Using a zero draft relieves some of the emotional pressure of writing a perfect product from the outset and provides the writer with some level of writing success for the day. At the end of a 30-minute period, a zero draft can go a long way to help the writer map out his or her ideas and identify how he or she wants to articulate thoughts in a first draft. A zero draft technique is also an effective way for the writer to identify gaps in his or her knowledge that he or she can further investigate prior to completing the first draft. A zero draft can be done on a computer or with paper and pencil depending on the writer's preference. For a conceptual topic, paper and pencil may be helpful for identifying connections between ideas. In these cases, concept maps or figures can be used to illustrate the flow of ideas as well. This approach may be particularly helpful for persons in the social sciences or any writer who is endeavoring to understand how concepts and constructs relate to each other, which can be helpful in creating a cohesive narrative or rhetorical argument.

Revision Process

Revisions are absolutely necessary in writing a completed scientific product.[4] Writers can be victim to a form of "tunnel vision" that results in not seeing simple mistakes within a scholarly product. Sometimes this becomes evident in small errors such as missing words or typos. Spellcheck programs are immensely helpful but cannot recognize that "regarding" is the word that was intended to be used within the sentence rather than "regrading." Both are spelled correctly but have different meanings and may leave the reader puzzled about the meaning of a sentence.

Conversely, another way that "writing tunnel vision" can be reflected in writing is when connections between thoughts and concepts within the product are not clearly expressed. It is important to remember that the reader may not have the same insight into the subject matter, and a writer may unwittingly omit information that is crucial for readers to understand links between

Sidebar 15-2

Below is an example of how a zero draft may look after a 20-minute writing session. In this case, the previously developed outline serves as a framework for the zero draft.

Outline—Yoga for the Treatment of Low Back Pain
1. Low Back Pain Prevalence/Incidence
   a. Burden of Low Back Pain on Society
   b. Financial Burden
   c. Quality of Life Changes
2. Treatment Options for Low Back Pain
3. Yoga as an Alternative Treatment Strategy

Zero Draft

Low back pain is a prevalent musculoskeletal injury with XX% of people in the US experiencing low back pain within their lifetime (find statistics to support and cite). Low back pain can affect people across multiple segments in the population and can be of particular concern in those that are physically active. (Find studies that support this idea and cite statistics of injury-related low back pain in physically active persons; NCAA study and RIO studies might be helpful here). The health care burden of low back pain is considerable. This includes financial costs for visits to primary care physicians, costs for medication, and therapeutic interventions for low back pain (find specific facts that identify costs of visits) in addition to the costs of time loss at work and physical activity. Low back pain can have deleterious effects on health-related quality of life. Multiple studies have shown that patients have concerns with impairments, activity limitations, and participation restrictions for a protracted period of time (be more specific and cite studies that demonstrate decreased quality of life through PROMs). In addition, multiple studies have identified that fear avoidance, kinesiophobia, and other psychosocial contextual factors also play a role in the resolution of low back pain.

Finding appropriate treatment strategies for low back pain is often difficult for clinicians given that, in many cases, the mechanical generator of low back pain cannot be identified. Multiple treatment algorithms and classifications systems have been proposed over the years to help provide direction. Some successful interventions for low back pain have included XX, XX, XX (need to find a systematic review; search the Cochrane database). XXXXX (Stuck here on how to make a transition about some of the potential limitations of the current low back pain treatment literature).

Yoga is an ancient practice that can include physical movement and postures, named *asanas*, with a focus on breath work and meditation. Yoga has gained popularity and approximately 13 million people practice some form of yoga in the United States (cite). Although yoga is typically used as a form of exercise, the benefits of yoga are both physical and mental (elaborate here on research in downregulation of the HPA axis and other physiological effects of yoga like stress reduction). Multiple, high-quality RCTs have been performed to examine the use of yoga as an intervention for low back pain and have found that yoga interventions lasting 4 to 6 weeks or longer significantly decrease pain and increase health-related quality of life (will need to expand here significantly with supporting citations and more data).

This next paragraph will focus on the yoga interventions and then will provide practical ways in which the athletic trainer can integrate some of these interventions into their clinical practice with athletes who are suffering from low back pain.

> **Sidebar 15-3**
>
> During the revision process, consider saving all forms of the electronic draft rather than saving over current work. As part of the naming convention for each file, include the date of the revised work so that you have a record of all the changes that have occurred in the paper. If you like to use Track Changes in a Word document, like I do, be sure that you save all changes in the final file before submitting the document. I have had students turn in work that includes edits that they did not realize were still present in the document because they were viewing the document via the "no mark-up" option in Track Changes.

ideas. Therefore, revisions are key to ensuring that writing is clear and conveys the thoughts that were intended.

To maximize the results of the revision process, the writer should expect to complete multiple drafts and build in the extra time to complete revisions accordingly. For example, a class paper that has a due date in 1 month should have a first draft completed at least 1 to 2 weeks in advance of the due date. To be able to revise with a clear mind, it is helpful for the writer to have some time between each series of revisions to be able to note problems with the paper. Putting a writing draft away for 24 hours allows the writer space and time to see the product clearly and with a critical eye. Viewing writing on a different medium may also prove to be helpful during the editing process. For example, printing out a paper and editing with a pen or pencil might be particularly helpful for some writers. Similarly, having someone else read a piece of writing can be valuable as long as the writer is ready to hear constructive criticism. The biggest mistake is for a writer to hide his or her writing. So much can be learned from an outsider's perspective. Knowing this, joining a writing circle or seeking the help of a professional at a university writing center may be a very helpful strategy (Sidebar 15-3).

Planning and Organization

Planning Process

Sometimes a writer may feel that time is a friend working in his or her favor or a foe threatening an impending deadline. A deadline is likely to produce some stress for a majority of writers. However, a deadline is a factor that is consistent and predictable in the writing process. Therefore, use the deadline as a starting point when trying to plan and organize the writing process. Grab a calendar and mark the due date for a project. Consider even creating an arbitrary deadline when one is not imposed. Once the deadline is identified, use a backward planning process to identify realistic writing goals leading back to the current date. Be sure to use the idea that writing is a process, so build into the identified writing goals multiple iterations of a document, manuscript, or chapter. Ideally, this is one of the first steps completed when planning. By planning early, what may seem like an overwhelming task can then be subdivided into "doable" chunks of work, leading to greater success and reducing stress. Recognize that, although much of the work on planning and organizing early in the writing process is important, it does not necessarily produce any tangible results. Nonetheless, this time spent planning is still important because it produces a roadmap for the writing project (Sidebar 15-4).

As part of the early planning process, the writer should also be clear about the purpose of the writing project and the intended audience.[5] Both the purpose of the writing project and intended audience shape the way that the scholarly product is crafted and influences tone, length, and style. Unless the writer is clear about the intended purpose and audience, he or she have to go back to make significant edits to the product, wasting time and increasing frustration. Some good ways to

Sidebar 15-4

There are a variety of ways to centralize article annotations or notes. As a student, my method of organizing notes was to read an article and organize information in a word document based on major concepts that I wanted to cover in my paper. Using the yoga and low back pain example in Sidebar 15-2, I could organize my notes using my outline as a guide. If I read an article that provided low back pain injury epidemiology data, I would paraphrase the information into a word document and cite the source. I would continue to do this for articles that I read and continue to add more information to each corresponding section of the outline. Similarly, if I read an article describing a randomized controlled trial of yoga in low back pain patients, I could summarize the findings (description of subjects, interventions, and findings) into the respective section of my outline. Once I finished creating annotations within each section of the outline, I was then prepared to start the writing process. I could use a zero draft to tie unifying ideas together in each section of my outline. From there, edits would then occur and, over a few writing sessions, my paper would really start to take shape.

understand the appropriate style and tone of a writing project is to read past examples. For example, when preparing a manuscript for submission to a journal, it is important to read other articles that have been published within that journal. Different fields of study also have different writing conventions, which can particularly influence manuscript styles and length. Similarly, for students completing a class writing project, a quick conversation with an instructor about the purpose of the writing project can help provide some additional direction for the writer.

Organization

Mise en place is a French culinary saying that literally means "everything in its place." *Mise en place* is a staple of busy kitchens because it allows chefs to consistently create a quality product in an efficient manner. Persons in the culinary industry essentially account for every minute of their time by creating lists of tasks that need to be done in a specific order over and over again. A chef's space is prepped, cleared of unnecessary clutter, and maximized for ergonomics to allow the chef to create a muscle memory of a task.

This philosophy can be applied to the writing process. This philosophy espouses the gathering and arranging of materials and tools needed for the writing tasks. A writer should organize his or her writing space with the items that he or she consistently reaches for, whether it be a pen to jot down notes or papers that are being used to reference. Similarly, the writer can organize documents on an electronic device so that annotations, notes, or references are easily found. Using the same methods consistently with writing will become a habit, and these habits can save valuable time when juggling multiple projects, as many students do. More importantly, by freeing up space in the brain for more complex tasks, the quality of thought processes may improve, leading to better writing.

Part of a *mise en place* philosophy is about focusing totally on the task at hand. A common pitfall for productive writing is that the writer becomes distracted by other things, people, or tasks. These distractions take away from the ability to make significant progress in writing and can derail a writer's progress toward a deadline. Common mistakes include allowing the flow of writing to be disrupted by phone calls, emails, social media posts, and conversations. Although it is important to take breaks from work on occasion, the activity from the break should not take too much mental energy or provide a persistent distraction once the break is over. This means that a writer must actually work against how he or she has been trained to work. Multitasking, an important skill, is one that should not necessarily be employed while working on writing. The

> ## Sidebar 15-5
>
> One of the biggest stressors that I have experienced as a graduate student is when I completed a paper only to find that my computer had a virus and that I had lost the whole document. I actually heard a colleague state that when she was in school, she had to type her dissertation on a typewriter. Imagine that! Given that it was her only physical copy of the dissertation, she would place her dissertation in the freezer at night because it was the safest place in a home if a fire occurred. Luckily, we have come a long way in being able to store multiple versions of work. The lesson in this is that having the right method to back up data and writing is imperative. There are many cost-effective ways that a student or professional can back up writing. Many use cloud-based storage. Regardless of the back-up strategy that is used, identify the strategy early and stick to it!

constant switching between tasks like flipping back between responding to an email and working on a paper requires a mental shift to be able to get back on task. For example, a study found that it takes 25 minutes to return to an original task after an interruption.[6] If a writer scheduled 1 hour for writing in a given day and has 2 task interruptions during that time period, then the writer has essentially completed approximately 10 minutes of truly focused writing. Wasted time adds up and then becomes a stressor as a deadline approaches.

There are a number of time sucks that can be sources of stress or can inadvertently cause stress by taking away from the time that a writer could be using toward making progress within his or her writing. One easy time suck to overcome is the time spent formatting and referencing a document. Reference management software is vital to saving precious time. Many universities now carry subscriptions to free reference-management software. Some of the software packages have a learning curve, but the time spent learning to use the software on the front end will save time on the back end of the writing process. Database searching can also prove to be a time suck when the writer does not keep track of his or her search process. Information to keep track of includes dates of searches, databases used, and successful uses of search terms. If not well managed, a writer may end up repeating searches and finding redundant information or miss some vital potential resources. Having an account with a database search engine like EBSCO is helpful because the account can be modified to keep track of a search history. It can also be programmed to create alerts and search folders. A reference librarian is a helpful resource in maximizing time spent completing database searches, particularly when learning to use Medical Subject Heading terms, Boolean searches, and search limits.

Another time suck during the writing process is spent in managing notes and annotations. As part of the organization process, each writer should develop a method for organizing notes related to research articles. Creating article annotations in a centralized document may be a helpful solution. The centralized document could contain essential information about each article including the research question, study design, variables measured, methodology, and results. In addition, annotations could contain some of the most salient findings and notes about how the article ties back to the writer's own scholarly project. Using the centralized annotations helps to avoid one common mistake that novice researchers make, which is to make notes regarding an article within the article (physical or electronic copy) only. When the writer then needs to sit down to synthesize thoughts and tie ideas together, he or she may have a hard time finding where a specific note about an article was written and could end up spending precious minutes trying to sift through a thick stack of articles to track down the correct article (Sidebar 15-5).

Conclusion

Writing stressors can be largely avoided if the writer understands that he or she may positively influence writing motivation, realizes that writing is a process that takes time to complete, and plans writing activities to maximize efficiency and minimize distractions. This common-sense approach to writing is intuitive but still requires practice and active engagement to do well. Thus, the saying by Johann Wolfgang von Goethe, "Knowing is not enough; we must apply. Willing is not enough; we must do" seems an apt perspective to take in creating an environment that enhances productivity and minimizes stress.

References

1. Troia GA, Shankland RK, Wolbers KA. Motivation research in writing: theoretical and empirical considerations. *Read Writ Q.* 2012;28:5-28.
2. Pajares F. Self-efficacy beliefs, motivation, and achievement in writing: a review of the literature. *Read Writ Q.* 2003;19:139-158.
3. Trimble JR. *Writing With Style.* 3rd ed. Boston, MA: Prentice Hall; 2011.
4. Lanham RA. *Revising Prose.* 2nd ed. New York, NY: MacMillan Publishing Company; 1987.
5. Kennedy AJ, Kennedy DM, Aaron JE. *The Bedford Reader.* 11th ed. Boston, MA: Bedford/St. Martins; 2012.
6. Mark G, Gudith D, Klocke U. The cost of interrupted work: more speed and stress. *Proc of CHI '08.* 2008:107-110.

Financial Disclosures

Dr. Rehal Bhojani has no financial or proprietary interest in the materials presented herein.

Dr. Craig R. Denegar has no financial or proprietary interest in the materials presented herein.

Dr. Jon Gray has no financial or proprietary interest in the materials presented herein.

Dr. Jay Hertel has no financial or proprietary interest in the materials presented herein.

Dr. Mark Knoblauch has no financial or proprietary interest in the materials presented herein.

Dr. Jeff G. Konin has no financial or proprietary interest in the materials presented herein.

Dr. Laura Kunkel has no financial or proprietary interest in the materials presented herein.

Dr. Mitzi S. Laughlin has no financial or proprietary interest in the materials presented herein.

Dr. Melissa Long has no financial or proprietary interest in the materials presented herein.

Dr. Thomas Lowder has no financial or proprietary interest in the materials presented herein.

Dr. Sarah A. Manspeaker has no financial or proprietary interest in the materials presented herein.

Dr. Jennifer M. Medina McKeon has no financial or proprietary interest in the materials presented herein.

Dr. Patrick O. McKeon has no financial or proprietary interest in the materials presented herein.

Dr. Elisabeth C. Rosencrum has no financial or proprietary interest in the materials presented herein.

Dr. Luzita Vela has no financial or proprietary interest in the materials presented herein.

Dr. Josh Yellen has no financial or proprietary interest in the materials presented herein.

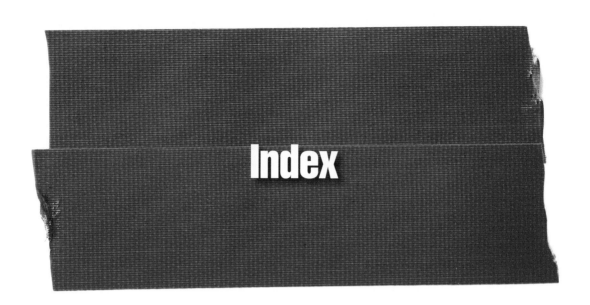

Index

Printed in the United States
by Baker & Taylor Publisher Services